Control of Cardiovascular Diseases in Developing Countries

Research, Development, and Institutional Strengthening

Committee on Research, Development, and Institutional
Strengthening for Control of Cardiovascular Diseases in
Developing Countries

Board on International Health

INSTITUTE OF MEDICINE

Christopher P. Howson, K. Srinath Reddy, Thomas J. Ryan, and
Judith R. Bale, *Editors*

NATIONAL ACADEMY PRESS
Washington, D.C.   1998

NATIONAL ACADEMY PRESS • 2101 Constitution Avenue, N.W. • Washington, D.C. 20418

NOTICE: The project that is the subject of this report was approved by the Governing Board of the National Research Council, whose members are drawn from the councils of the National Academy of Sciences, the National Academy of Engineering, and the Institute of Medicine. The members of the committee responsible for the report were chosen for their special competences and with regard for appropriate balance.

The Institute of Medicine was chartered in 1970 by the National Academy of Sciences to enlist distinguished members of the appropriate professions in the examination of policy matters pertaining to the health of the public. In this, the Institute acts under both the Academy's 1863 congressional charter responsibility to be an adviser to the federal government and its own initiative in identifying issues of medical care, research, and education. Dr. Kenneth I. Shine is president of the Institute of Medicine.

This study was supported by the World Health Organization. The views presented in this report are those of the Institute of Medicine Committee on Research, Development, and Institutional Strengthening for Control of Cardiovascular Diseases in Developing Countries and are not necessarily those of the funding organization.

International Standard Book No. 0-309-06137-7

Additional copies of this report are available for sale from the National Academy Press, Box 285, 2101 Constitution Avenue, N.W., Washington, DC 20055. Call (800) 624-6242 or (202) 334-3313 (in the Washington metropolitan area), or visit the NAP's on-line bookstore at: **www.nap.edu**.

The full text of this report is available on line at: **www.nap.edu/readingroom.**

For more information about the Institute of Medicine, visit the IOM home page at: **www2.nas.edu/iom**.

The serpent has been a symbol of long life, healing, and knowledge among almost all cultures and religions since the beginning of recorded history. The image adopted as a logotype by the Institute of Medicine is based on a relief carving from ancient Greece, now held by the Staatliche Museen in Berlin.

iv

HEATHER CALLAHAN, Administrative/Research Assistant (until February 1998)
STACEY KNOBLER, Administrative/Research Assistant (after April 1998)
SHARON GALLOWAY, Financial Associate

♦ ♦ ♦ ♦ ♦ ♦

Preface

Cardiovascular diseases (CVDs) are increasing in epidemic proportions in developing countries. Of the 52 million deaths reported worldwide in 1990, 15 million were attributable to CVD (World Bank, 1993). CVD already accounts for almost 10 percent of the total global burden of disease and most likely became the developing world's leading cause of death in the mid-1990s.

There is reason for hope, however, given that huge potential exists for applying R&D to prevention or control of the emerging epidemic. It is frequently noted that half of all the gains in human life expectancy of the past several thousand years have occurred in this century. As the report of the Ad Hoc Committee on Health Research points out, although some of these gains have resulted directly from improvements in economic and educational standards, another important factor is the advance in scientific knowledge and its application both in creating powerful new interventions such as vaccines and dietary supplements and in guiding behavior (Ad Hoc Committee, 1996). If one assumes that growth in scientific knowledge will continue to be of fundamental importance, investments in health research will help prevent, and control health problems and protect the health benefits that result from socioeconomic development. This can vastly improve health and economic productivity, particularly for CVDs which are so amenable to intervention.

In addition, a considerable body of evidence suggests that current programs for CVD risk factor prevention and low-cost case management offer feasible, cost-effective ways to reduce CVD mortality and disability in developing country populations (Pearson et al., 1993). In most developing countries, however, implementation of these programs is hampered by the lack of awareness of these options. The view that investments in CVD detract from investments in communicable disease control and childhood, maternal, and reproductive health reflects an unfortunate competition among opportunities for improving health. Clearly, the latter remain a high priority, but each investment needs to be evaluated according to its costs and benefits.

Although control of communicable, childhood, and maternal diseases has benefited from several decades of international efforts in epidemiology, clinical care, policy, and implementation, such large-scale efforts for CVD are lacking and have left both governments and individuals to make choices about health and health care services without adequate information on the costs and benefits of the alternatives. There remains, therefore, an increasing need to promote policy dialogue on CVD and to base this dialogue on informed knowledge of R&D opportunities in CVD that offer effective, affordable, and widely applicable responses in developing countries.

PROJECT CHARGE

This project was designed to provide such a basis for the work of the Global Forum for Health Research, a newly formed international organization of governments of low- and middle-income countries, major traditional "donors," and health researchers. The task of the Forum, which met for the first time in June 1997, is to assess R&D opportunities for solving health problems in developing countries and to identify the flow of resources to meet these needs. The Forum also convinces governments and other investors of the benefits of health research in improving health and enhancing economic development among the poorest populations. To function effectively, the Forum requires access to (1) high-quality data on disease burden; (2) reasons for the persistence of this burden; (3) measurements of the cost-effectiveness of potential interventions; (4) estimates of current patterns of spending on R&D; and (5) assessments of national health systems. It thus requested that the Institute of Medicine (IOM) of the U.S. National Academy of Sciences prepare a report with appropriate data for CVD.

To accomplish this task, the IOM constituted an international committee of 13 members representing broad expertise in clinical cardiology; epidemiology and research methods, including clinical trials; international health and R&D policy; health economics; traditional medicine; and nutrition as they relate to CVD prevention and control. Special attention was given to obtaining the input of developing countries, through committee membership, consultations with expert groups, and developing country experts on the Academy panel that provided independent peer review of the committee's report. In addition, 11 liaison members with appropriate expertise and institutional affiliations assisted the committee by providing information at initial deliberations and by commenting on preliminary reports. Although liaison members provided important information and perspective, the report findings and recommendations are those of the primary committee alone.

An initial three-hour meeting of the committee was held in conjunction with the Fourth International Conference on Preventive Cardiology in Montreal. Members in attendance agreed on the key issues to be addressed, an outline for the report, and author assignments for first drafts of chapters. A number of committee members, liaisons, and staff also participated in a symposium on June 30, 1997, organized by Arun Chockalingam of the Canadian Coalition for High Blood Pressure Prevention and Control and Prabhat Jha of the World Bank, and cochaired by Darwin Labarthe of the University of Texas-Houston School of Public Health and Fred Paccaud of the Institut Universitaire de Médicine Sociale et Préventive of Lausanne. The symposium provided an important starting point for the part of the committee's report dealing with institutional arrangements in support of CVD R&D. The full committee then met on November 13–14, 1997, to review the report draft and identify needs for revision. The committee's report underwent independent peer review in February–May 1998.

ORGANIZATION OF THE REPORT

This report contains six chapters, an epilogue, and two appendixes in addition to the summary chapter. Chapters 1 and 2 describe the current and future burden of CVD in developing countries. Chapter 3 describes current practices in CVD prevention and care in developing countries, and Chapter 4 reports the findings of a committee survey to determine the levels and types of R&D that currently support CVD prevention and treatment in developing countries. Chapter 5 summarizes the needs, opportunities, and priorities for global R&D. Chapter 6 outlines recommended institutional arrangements under which these activities can best be facilitated and enhanced, and the Epilogue comments on the question: Why should countries in the developed world care about the emerging epidemic of CVD in developing countries? Appendix A presents the rationale for the committee's recommendations according to the five-step procedure for setting priorities in health research proposed in the Ad Hoc Committee's report. Appendix B provides a glossary of terms.

The committee offers this report to help educate funders, health policymakers, and the medical community about the emerging epidemic of CVD in developing countries and the threat it poses to countries least able to afford it. More importantly, this report recommends R&D opportunities and priorities to reduce CVD in developing countries. It is hoped that these can assist the Forum and other funders to direct funding to the support of scientifically robust, coherent R&D that complements other public health initiatives.

K. Srinath Reddy and Thomas J. Ryan, *Cochairs*

◆ ◆ ◆ ◆ ◆

Acknowledgments

The committee is grateful to the many individuals who contributed to this report. In particular, it thanks Prabhat Jha for providing substantive background for the study; Arun Chockalingam, Kathleen Dracup, William Harlan, Christopher Howson, Prabhat Jha, Thomas Pearson, and Srinath Reddy for their chapter drafts; and Liu Lisheng, Walinjom Muna, Il Suh, and Magdi Yacoub for their substantive contributions to the committee deliberations. The committee expresses its appreciation to Fred Paccaud fororganizing an initial meeting of implementers around the committee's charge and for his input to the next stages of the project. The committee thanks its liaison members for their essential contributions to the project and the following reviewers for their substantive input into the report: Ximena Berrios, WHO–Interhealth Project, Santiago; A.O. Falase, University of Ibadan Teaching Hospital, Ibadan, Il Soon Kim, Yonsei University College of Medicine, Seoul; Jean Claude Mbanya, University of Yaoundé I, Yaoundé; Rafael G. Oganov, Cardiology Research Center, Moscow; Munro H. Proctor, Boston University School of Medicine, Boston; and Cheira Suporrsilaphachai, Ministry of Public Health, Bangkok.

The committee is grateful to the following institutions for providing information on current and projected CVD funding flows: Australian Agency for International Development, Australia; Victorian Health Promotion Foundation, Australia; Federal Chancellery, Austria; Secrétaire d'Etat à la Coopération adjoint au Premier Ministre, Belgium; Canadian International Development Agency, Canada; Ministry of Foreign Affairs, Denmark; European Commission, Belgium; Ministry of Foreign Affairs, Finland; Ministre délégué de la Coopération et du Développement, France; Bundesministerium für Wirtschaftliche Zusammenarbeit und Entwicklung, Germany; Department of Foreign Affairs, Ireland; Ministry of Foreign Affairs, Italy; Ministry of Foreign Affairs, Japan;

Secrétaire d'état pour les Affaires étrangères, Commerce extérieur et Coopération, Luxembourg; Ministry for Development Cooperation, Netherlands; Ministry of Foreign Affairs and Trade, New Zealand; Royal Ministry of Foreign Affairs, Norway; Instituto da Cooperaçao Portuguesa (I.C.P.), Portugal; Ministère
des Affaires étrangères, France; Ministry of Foreign Affairs, Sweden; Départe-
ment Fédéral des Affaires étrangères, Switzerland; Overseas Development Ad-
ministration, United Kingdom; Agency for International Development, United
States; Carnegie Corporation of New York, United States; Kaiser Family Foundation, United States; and the National Institutes of Health, United States.

The committee thanks the IOM staff—Heather Callahan, Stacey Knobler,
Sharon Galloway, Mike Edington, and Claudia Carl—for their essential roles in
the project. The cochairs thank Judith Bale for her role in completing the final
drafts and Christopher Howson for his effective leadership and strong commitment to CVD prevention and control in the developing world.

Finally, the committee wishes to note the following special contributors:
Dean Jamison for his vision for the project and persistence in securing support
for the study, Prabhat Jha for his inestimable assistance with key sections of the
report, Darwin Labarthe for his keen editorial eye and substantive contributions
during report review, and Srinath Reddy and Thomas Ryan for their effective
leadership of this fast-track project.

This project was funded by the World Health Organization. The committee
is deeply appreciative of its support and of the commitment and productive efforts of Tore Godal and Thomas Nchinda.

This report has been reviewed by individuals chosen for their diverse per-
spectives and technical expertise, in accordance with procedures approved by the
National Research Council's Report Review Committee. The purpose of this
independent review is to provide candid and critical comments that will assist the
authors and the IOM in making the published report as sound as possible and to
ensure that the report meets institutional standards for objectivity, evidence, and
responsiveness to the study charge. The content of the review comments and the
draft manuscript remain confidential to protect the integrity of the deliberative
process. We wish to thank the following individuals for their participation in the
review process: Francois Abboud, University of Iowa College of Medicine; John
Chalmers, Royal North Shore Hospital, St. Leonards, Australia; Chen Chun-
ming, Chinese Academy of Preventive Medicine, Beijing; Shanta C. Emmanuel,
Ministry of Health, Singapore; and A.D. Mbewu, South Africa Medical Research
Council, Cape Town. Although the individuals acknowledged have provided
valuable comments and suggestions, responsibility for the final content of this
report rests solely with the authoring committee and the IOM.

◆ ◆ ◆ ◆ ◆

Contents

Control of Cardiovascular Diseases in Developing Countries

◆ ◆ ◆ ◆ ◆ ◆

Executive Summary

Over the last century, life expectancy at birth has, for most populations, increased by more than 25 years. The epidemiologic transition, described more than 20 years ago, is key to understanding this global improvement in health and planning for future improvements (Omran, 1971). The transition recognizes, primarily because of the aging population worldwide, that the spectrum of disease in developing countries is changing from one of communicable diseases and perinatal and nutritional disorders to one of predominantly noncommunicable disease, most notably cardiovascular disease (CVD). This is the term used by the scientific community to embrace not just conditions of the heart (coronary artery disease; valvular, muscular, and congenital disease), but also hypertension and conditions involving the cerebral, carotid, and peripheral circulation. This report addresses the research needed to improve understanding of the scope of this challenge, the various risk factors involved, and ways of preventing and treating these diseases that will be both feasible and affordable for the developing world.

CVD has been identified as the primary noncommunicable health problem throughout the developing world. This is so for a number of reasons. The contribution of CVD to the burden of disease is increasing, all socioeconomic groups are vulnerable, and CVD inflicts major economic and human costs. Of the 52 million deaths reported worldwide in 1990, 15 million are attributable to CVD. CVD accounts for almost 10 percent of the global burden of disease measured by a combination of death and disability, and this is expected to increase to nearly 15 percent by the year 2020. By the mid-1990s, CVD most likely became the developing world's leading cause of death. It is not surprising, therefore, that a recent report of the Ad Hoc Committee on Health and Research refers to CVD as an "emerging epidemic" (Ad Hoc Committee, 1996). On a global scale, the two principal forms of CVD are ischemic heart disease and cerebrovascular dis-

1

ease (stroke), which together account for two-thirds of the CVD burden; the projected increase in total CVD burden is largely attributable to these conditions. Data on the economic cost of CVD in developing countries are limited, but in the United States, the direct and indirect costs of CVD are already 3 percent of the gross national product. In developing countries, CVD is more likely to attack adults in their productive middle years than it is in developed countries. This has a profound and adverse impact on households, families, and society.

What explanation can be offered for the global epidemic of CVD and the expectation that it will worsen in the future?

• The world population is expanding by 80 million people per year. Because of declining mortality and fertility rates, this increase is most notable among the middle- and older-age groups that are likely to develop CVD.

• Economic development has brought higher incomes that are allowing the adoption of a Western life-style, which may include a diet high in fat, sugar, and salt; increased tobacco use; and less physical activity. These behavioral changes have been accelerated by rapid migration of large populations to the major cities of developing countries.

• Interactions among risk factors can increase the incidence of CVD. The impact of adopting a Western life-style can be severe when more than one behavior change predisposes to CVD.

Given the enormous potential for applying research and technological advances to prevention and treatment of CVD, there is hope that the epidemic can be controlled. The following observations suggest that premature death can be avoided and the quality of life improved in middle and later years:

• dramatic declines in CVD mortality in Western countries;
• geographic variations in CVD mortality; and
• established associations of adult mortality with modifiable risk factors, such as tobacco use and obesity.

Reducing the prevalence of CVD risk factors has been shown to decrease mortality and disability in middle-aged and older persons and to lead to a better quality of life. Risk factor prevention programs and low-cost case management are feasible, cost-effective ways of reducing CVD mortality and disability.

In most developing countries, however, implementation of these approaches and programs is hampered by the lack of awareness of cost-effective CVD control options and the concern that investment in CVD will detract from efforts to control communicable diseases and improve perinatal and nutritional disorders. It is important, therefore, to develop a dialogue based on informed understanding of the growing threat that CVD poses to developing countries and of the need for research and development (R&D) to provide effective, affordable, and widely applicable responses to this threat.

This Institute of Medicine (IOM) report provides a basis for the dialogue. It offers recommendations on opportunities and priorities for R&D to reduce the CVD burden in developing countries, as well as the institutional arrangements needed to achieve these goals. The IOM committee approached its assessment of the scope of the problem by following the five-step sequence proposed in the Ad Hoc Committee's report: (1) determine the size of the CVD burden, (2) identify the reasons for the CVD burden, (3) evaluate the adequacy of the current knowledge base, (4) evaluate the promise of R&D efforts, and (5) assess the adequacy of the current level of effort. This rationale is described further in Appendix A.

RECOMMENDATIONS

The committee used the following four criteria to establish priorities for R&D investment to control CVD in developing countries:

1. Investments should have a large-scale impact on populations, regardless of gender, socioeconomic status, or geographic location. Incremental implementation of investments may be necessary in many countries.

2. Investments in one country should involve methods and processes (but not necessarily results) that are broadly transferable to other low- and middle-income countries.

3. Investments should yield results within a time frame of 5 to 10 years, although evaluation of the results over a longer term may be desirable.

4. Investments should focus on measurable data with collection that follows established methodologies in epidemiology, health policy, economics, and social behavior.

Using these criteria, the committee prepared recommendations for R&D investment in six broad areas for the control of CVD:

1. Determine the magnitude of the CVD burden in developing countries.

2. Develop targeted, effective primordial and primary prevention strategies using case-control studies.

3. Reduce tobacco use.

4. Detect and treat high blood pressure.

5. Initiate pilot studies to evaluate essential vascular packages of effective, low-cost drugs.

6. Develop and assess algorithms of affordable clinical care for CVD.

To support the first six recommendations, the committee then recognized broader needs with two additional recommendations:

7. Build the capacity to conduct R&D activities.

8. Develop institutional mechanisms that facilitate CVD prevention and control.

Determine the Magnitude of the CVD Burden in Developing Countries

Recommendation 1. Create standardized surveys using networks such as the MONICA (World Health Organization Multinational *Moni*toring of Trends and Determinants in *Ca*rdiovascular Disease) model (including selected sentinel sites) to monitor levels and trends of clinical events and cardiovascular risk factors.

The major goal of these surveys is to describe the prevalence and distribution of clinical events and of conventional risk factors associated with CVD by age, sex, and ethnicity in representative samples of the population. Thus, the surveys should involve moderately large sample sizes (several tens of thousands or hundreds of thousands of people) and simple, focused data collection activities. Like vital registration, cross-sectional surveys of this type require a valid sampling frame. Ideally, data from local cross-sectional studies should be linked to local estimates of the magnitude of various risk factors, which would be drawn from case-control or prospective studies. Survey data could also be linked to local mortality data.

The recommended surveys should be repeated at regular intervals to assess trends in the levels and distribution of CVD risk factors. If the surveys are appropriately designed to allow repeated observations of many individuals and to take successive independent samples, they can also be used to quantify the strength of association between a CVD risk factor with eventual development of disease. However, patient follow-up in many developing country populations is difficult because of a lack of vital registration systems, high population mobility, and variable access to medical care. Thus, it may be easier in such populations to classify mortality status rather than attempt to record nonfatal events associated with CVD.

Recommendation 2. Expand national and regional systems for vital registration.

There are several ways to obtain essential vital registration information. The essential information is a record of *all* deaths in the population, classified by age and sex. Priority assistance should be given to countries that currently lack a system to obtain this basic information. Appropriate sampling frames should be built into each system to allow identification of geographic, ethnic, and rural and urban differences in CVD mortality and morbidity.

In developing countries, most vital registries are government funded and lack a research component. Where registration systems are currently inadequate improved systems must be developed. One possibility is the capture–recapture method for deriving better estimates of total deaths.

Recommendation 3. Improve the accuracy and completeness of cause-of-death statistics.

Cause-of-death studies, which provide information on the underlying reasons for death, currently exist only in developed countries and, to a lesser extent, in Latin America. Determination of cause-specific mortality in most developing countries could be strengthened through the use of community-based random samples, sentinel sites, surveillance systems modeled after those used in the MONICA model, and verbal autopsy techniques (i.e., techniques that involve questioning relatives in person or by phone about the circumstances surrounding a death, especially for CVD-related deaths). Thus, priority areas for research support are establishing and evaluating sentinel registration sites, and validating and using verbal autopsy techniques.

Recommendation 4. Develop better estimates of disability.

Most developing countries lack reliable estimates of the level of disability caused by CVD or other diseases. Further, the estimates that are available are not standardized across populations. Focused pilot studies could generate appropriate estimates with standard, validated measures of quality-of-life.

Develop Targeted, Effective Primordial and Primary Prevention Strategies Using Case-Control Studies

Recommendation 5. Determine the contributions to morbidity and mortality of established and new risk factors for CVD, and assess their interactions with case-control studies.

Case-control studies of disease incidence can identify the strength of association between a risk factor and CVD. They may also uncover new risk factors. Although prospective studies are more robust methodologically because exposure to the risk factor demonstrably precedes disease, retrospective case-control studies can usually generate needed data more quickly and at lower cost. Ideally, the occurrence of first myocardial infarctions should be studied to avoid survival bias and postmorbid modification of risk factors. Key conditions that might be studied using case-control methods include acute myocardial infarction, acute stroke, transient ischemic attacks, congestive heart failure, and peripheral vascular disease. Established risk factors for CVD include hypertension, tobacco use, dietary intakes high in fat, salt, and sugar, and inadequate exercise.

Reduce Tobacco Use

Recommendation 6. Research on tobacco control in developing countries should (1) estimate the prevalence of regular tobacco use in population samples; (2) monitor tobacco consumption trends in vulnerable groups such as children, adolescents, and women; (3) evaluate the cost-effectiveness of community-based interventions that promote abstinence from tobacco; (4) evaluate the cost-effectiveness of tobacco cessation programs aimed at changing the behavior of current smokers; and (5) estimate the economic impact of tobacco control on developing countries that grow and manufacture tobacco or tobacco products for domestic or foreign markets in order to encourage the change to alternative crops and manufacturing.

Current levels of risk factors, most notably tobacco usage, will determine future age-specific mortality and morbidity rates. The numbers of global deaths and of disability-adjusted life years (DALYs) that result from tobacco use are expected to increase to about 8.3 million and 124 million, respectively, by 2020, with more than 70 percent of these occurring in developing countries. These trends amount to a doubling of the percentage of current deaths due to tobacco use worldwide and a tripling of current DALYs lost. Thus, decreasing tobacco use would reduce both the substantial burden of CVD-associated disease projected for developing countries and the significant burden of other tobacco-related diseases, including certain cancers and chronic obstructive pulmonary disease.

Detect and Treat High Blood Pressure

Recommendation 7. Research on the control of hypertension in developing country populations should be undertaken to (1) estimate the distribution of high blood pressure and the prevalence of hypertension in populations; (2) evaluate the cost-effectiveness of community-based, life-style-linked interventions (salt intake, increase exercise, improve stress management) aimed at decreasing the incidence of high blood pressure; (3) assess the cost-effectiveness of programs to detect and treat hypertension by improving awareness, treatment initiation and adherence, and level of control; and (4) evaluate the effectiveness of low-cost combination drug therapies developed by countries such as China.

High blood pressure is a major contributor to both coronary heart disease and stroke. Even small decreases in the incidence of high blood pressure could have a profound effect on lowering CVD rates. Hypertension control programs are an ideal first step for CVD prevention and control for a number of reasons: (1) hypertension is a risk factor for both coronary heart disease and stroke; (2) such programs have a "clinical" appeal to both care providers and the community; (3) the results are easily measurable; (4) the impact on hypertension awareness, treatment status, and level of control can be measured in a relatively short time (i.e., five years); (5) such programs create a natural coalition among various categories of health care providers (nurses, multipurpose health workers, general practitioners, internists, cardiologists, nephrologists, neurologists, obstetricians, ophthalmologists, nutritionists, stress therapists, and exercise program managers) who play an important role in the detection or management of hypertension and its sequelae; and (6) the concept of "comprehensive cardiovascular reduction" as part of hypertension management makes it possible to incorporate strategies aimed at modifying other CVD risk factors, such as tobacco use, high blood lipid levels, diabetes, and obesity.

Initiate Pilot Studies to Evaluate Essential Vascular Packages of Effective, Low-Cost Drugs

Recommendation 8. Evaluate the responses of different ethnic populations to cardiovascular drugs and interventions, and determine whether any different responses have implications for drug treatment.

Recommendation 9. Expand the participation of developing country research institutions in multicenter, collaborative clinical trials of essential vascular packages (EVPs) and other affordable, widely applicable interventions.

Evidence from randomized trials indicates that several of the clinical treatments now available can provide cost-effective care for patients with established CVD. Aspirin, beta-blockers, angiotensin-converting enzyme inhibitors, and cholesterol-lowering statin drugs reduce the probability of death and subsequent nonfatal major vascular events in patients with established ischemic heart disease. However, to have a sustained impact in developing countries, these drugs will have to be inexpensive and widely accessible. Although cholesterol-lowering drugs such as statins are currently expensive compared to aspirin or beta-blockers, their costs may decrease in the next five years when their patents expire. These drugs could then become key components of an EVP, or combination of drugs, that would be used to treat patients with CVD. The committee believes strongly that large numbers of people in developing countries could benefit from such an EVP. Because its delivery would rely on patients presenting themselves for treatment and would not involve screening costs, the EVP could be highly cost-effective. Packaging EVPs into single, once-a-day formulations, as is done for multidrug treatment of tuberculosis, could substantially improve compliance.

The goals for the EVP should be (1) to use low-cost, generic versions of drugs; (2) to achieve near-universal access to these proven interventions; and (3) to price the packages so they are affordable for developing country clinics and patients. The acceptability, use, and effectiveness of the EVP will have to be assessed, along with other parameters that measure diffusion into practice (discussed under Recommendation 10). Such testing could be in the form of randomized trials assessing delivery of the package versus standard clinical care. If acceptable, the EVP should then be included both in a publicly financed, universally available essential package of clinical services and in treatment lists covered by health insurance. Efforts to educate physicians and to increase patient awareness about the value of such packages should also be supported. Goals (2) and (3) could be addressed by pricing the reimbursements for treatment to the lowest-cost basis of the EVP.

Develop and Assess Algorithms of Affordable Clinical Care for CVD

Recommendation 10. Research should be undertaken to develop algorithms for affordable diagnosis and management of hypertension, dyslipidemia, diabetes, acute myocardial infarction, angina, stroke, transient ischemic attacks, congestive heart failure, peripheral vascular disease, post-myocardial infarction rehabilitation and risk management, and poststroke rehabilitation and risk management.

The development of algorithms for CVD care could improve the awareness and utilization of effective treatments. To be maximally effective, the algorithms should be adapted to address different cultural needs and should be widely applicable and usable by both physicians and nonphysicians and for different levels of care. Each algorithm should define clinical diagnostic or presumptive criteria, along with the steps for administering and evaluating simple medical treatments.

The acceptability and use of each algorithm should be measured, appropriate marketing developed for both the public and private sectors, and cooperation obtained from the pharmaceutical industry. The algorithms should be developed and implemented according to local needs and cultural norms. Further, the results of using an algorithm for CVD care should be monitored and the impact on disease outcome evaluated.

Build the Capacity to Conduct R&D Activities

Recommendation 11. Building regional capacity for R&D requires establishing or expanding: (1) training programs in cardiovascular epidemiology, clinical research methodology, health policy research, and health economics; (2) institutional capacity for undertaking integrated research relevant to CVD control; and (3) collaboration through twin-center programs and regional research networks.

The capacity to conduct research at regional and local levels must be strengthened before efforts to control CVD can be effective in developing countries. Therefore, the level and intensity of training in public health and preventive medicine have to be substantially increased throughout the developing world, not just for highly educated health professionals but, more important, for health workers at all levels. Only a small fraction of the necessary training capacity can be achieved through existing programs and methods; further, even the current capacity cannot be maintained without vigorous continuing education programs. For the recommendations in this report to be implemented productively in developing countries, a major international commitment must be made for the development of training programs and the use of current technologies. These are needed to improve the effectiveness of efforts and investments in CVD control.

Develop Institutional Mechanisms for Facilitating CVD Prevention and Control

Recommendation 12. The committee recommends establishing a Steering Committee for CVD R&D under the aegis of the Global Forum for Health Research. The functions of this committee would include, but not be limited to, the following: (1) establishing a program of competitive grant awards in priority areas of CVD research, modeled after the United Nations Development Programme–World Bank–World Health Organization Special Programme for Research and Training in Tropical Diseases; (2) establishing a global network on CVD health policy; and (3) promoting exchanges of CVD scientists from industry, academia, and the ministries of developing and developed countries.

It has become increasingly important to consider the organizational arrangements that will facilitate CVD prevention and control around the world. The ultimate goal is to establish an R&D capability that will be effective and sustainable. The committee's recommendation for creating a Steering Committee for Cardiovascular R&D stresses flexibility in priority setting, competitive grant making, and global networking and partnering. These characteristics are hall-marks of the Special Programme for Research and Training in Tropical Diseases and led to its selection as the model for the proposed steering committee.

The control of communicable, childhood, and maternal diseases worldwide has benefited from several decades of major international efforts. Such large-scale efforts are lacking for CVD. Yet the evidence that premature death can be avoided and quality of life improved in later years includes dramatic declines in CVD mortality in Western countries, geographic variation in CVD mortality, and established associations of adult mortality with modifiable risk factors, such as tobacco use and obesity. Reducing the prevalence of these risk factors has been shown to decrease mortality in both middle-aged and older persons and to lead to less disability and a better quality of life in later years. Programs for risk factor prevention and low-cost case management of CVD offer feasible, cost-effective ways to reduce CVD mortality and disability in developing countries. They should yield high payoffs in health status and in economic productivity.

1

♦ ♦ ♦ ♦ ♦

The Current Burden of Cardiovascular Diseases in Developing Countries

ECONOMIC DEVELOPMENT BRINGS CHANGES

Although cardiovascular diseases (CVDs) are well known throughout the world, their form and the burden they cause change as a country undergoes economic development. Developing countries begin with a disease burden dominated by nutritional, perinatal, and infectious diseases and, in the process of development, make the transition to one dominated by noncommunicable diseases, particularly CVD (Olshansky and Ault, l986; Omram, 1971). The four stages of that transition are shown in Table 1-1.

For countries in the earliest stage of development, the predominant circulatory diseases are rheumatic heart disease (Box 1-1), infections, and nutritional deficiency-related disorders of the heart muscle. Regions in this phase include Sub-Saharan Africa and the rural areas of South America and Asia. In the second stage, as infectious disease burdens are reduced and nutrition improves, diseases related to hypertension, such as hemorrhagic stroke (Box 1-2) and hypertensive heart disease (Box 1-3), become more common. Regions in this phase include China and other Asian countries. In the third stage, as life expectancy continues to improve, high-fat diets, cigarette smoking, and sedentary life-styles become more common. Noncommunicable diseases then predominate, with the highest mortality caused by atherosclerotic CVD, most frequently ischemic heart disease and atherothrombotic stroke, especially at ages of less than 50 years. This phase is found in urban India (Reddy and Yusuf, 1998) and the former socialist countries including Russia. In the fourth stage, increased efforts to prevent, diagnose, and treat ischemic heart disease and stroke are able to delay the impact of these diseases to more advanced ages. The regions that have reached this final stage are Western Europe, North America (excluding Mexico), Australia, and New Zealand.

11

TABLE 1-1 Deaths Caused by Cardiovascular Disease at Different Stages of Development—1990

Stage of Development	Deaths from CVD (% of total)	Predominant CVDs	Regional Examples
Age of pestilence and famine	5–10	Rheumatic heart disease, infections, and nutritional cardiomyopathies	Sub-Saharan Africa, rural India, and South America
Age of receding pandemics	10–35	As above, plus hypertensive heart disease and hemorrhagic stroke	China
Age of degenerative and man-made diseases	35–55	All forms of stroke; ischemic heart disease at relatively young ages	Urban India, formerly socialist economies
Age of delayed degenerative diseases	<50	Stroke and ischemic heart disease at older ages	Western Europe. North America, Australia, New Zealand

SOURCE: Jha et al., forthcoming.

BOX 1-1 Rheumatic Heart Disease: The Unfinished Agenda

For countries in the early stages of development, rheumatic heart disease is the most common form of CVD. Indeed, it is thought to affect more than 4 million people worldwide, resulting in approximately 90,000 deaths each year (Michaud et al., 1993). It is caused by group A streptococcal pharyngitis, which if untreated will progress in about 3 percent of cases to rheumatic fever and then cause immunologic damage to heart valves and muscle. Many years later, the thickened or incompetent heart valves disrupt blood flow, which leads to congestive heart failure or death. Although rheumatic fever and rheumatic heart disease have essentially disappeared in developed countries, both remain major causes of CVD in developing countries. In Africa, Latin America, Asia (especially India), and the Pacific Islands, 1–2 percent of school children show evidence of rheumatic valvular disease (Michaud et al., 1993). A high proportion of these children will develop progressive heart failure over the next 20–40 years, then die at 25 to 44 years of age. A range of 20–35 percent of cardiac patients admitted to hospitals in Africa and Asia have rheumatic heart disease, often with heart failure or needing replacement of the heart valve. This surgery is effective at prolonging life, but where it is not available, referrals abroad are costly. For the next 20–40 years, it is likely that developing countries will experience a double burden of CVD: rheumatic heart disease will continue, while atherosclerotic CVD becomes more common.

For most developing and middle-income countries, the increased incidence of CVD adds to the continuing burden of infectious, nutritional, and perinatal diseases. It is a major setback for health care systems that are already overburdened and underfunded (WHO, 1997, Box 1-4).

Subsets of a population may be at different stages of the CVD epidemic. An "early-adopter" community such as one with rapid social and economic development may experience an early increase in CVD and thus have a higher level than other parts of the population. The decline in CVD burden may also occur earlier for this community, as shown in Figure 1-1. The transition of CVD from a disease of the wealthy to one of the poor has been documented in the United Kingdom and the United States (Kaplan and Keil, 1993; Marmot et al., 1991). It was relatively rare in the African-American community in the 1960s, but now its incidence equals or exceeds that in the white population of the United States (NHLBI, 1996). The pattern of disease continues to be in transition for all but the most developed countries.

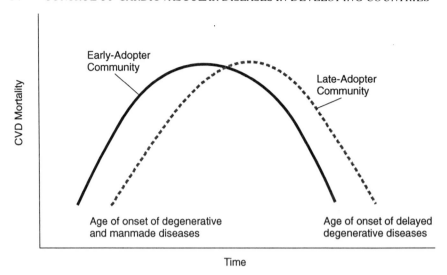

FIGURE 1-1 Theoretical comparison of cardiovascular disease mortality in early- versus late-adopter communities.

ATHEROSCLEROSIS AS THE UNDERLYING DISEASE PROCESS

Vital statistics and hospital admission records show the clinical syndromes of myocardial infarction, sudden cardiac death, atherothrombotic stroke, and peripheral arterial disease to be the leading causes of morbidity and mortality. These diseases share the same pathology, atherosclerosis. This disease process is thought to begin in adolescence with injury to the arterial endothelium and focal accumulation of lipid-filled macrophages known as fatty streaks. These lesions are common worldwide. Some fatty streaks progress by infiltration and proliferation of smooth muscle cells to form the fibrous-capped plaque characteristic of atherosclerosis. The plaques appear to be less common in developing countries. They are clinically silent until the fourth decade of life, when they undergo fissuring, ulceration, and thrombosis, leading to the clinical syndromes of ischemic heart disease, stroke, and peripheral vascular disease. Although the manifestation differs with the artery involved, the clinical syndromes are all related to the same systemic disease process, atherosclerosis (Ross, 1993) (see Appendix B for further discussion of clinical syndromes).

Risk Factors for Atherosclerotic Disease

The risk factors associated with atherosclerotic disease include demographic, familial, behavioral, and physiological characteristics. The roles of many of these factors in the pathophysiology of atherosclerosis have been defined (Fuster et al., 1996). They can be classified on the basis of whether they are modifiable (Pasternak et al., 1996; Pearson et al., 1993) (Figure 1-2). Nonmodifiable risk factors include age, male gender, and a positive family history of CVD with onset at an early age. Modifiable risk factors can be behavioral (sedentary life-style, a diet high in fat and cholesterol, cigarette smoking) or physiological (elevated low-density lipoprotein [LDL] cholesterol, decreased high-density lipoprotein [HDL] cholesterol, diabetes, hypertension, obesity, postmenopausal status [in women]). The effectiveness of modifying risk factors to prevent disease has been dramatic for some risk factors. For others, the association with atherosclerotic disease is less well understood (see Appendix B).

BOX 1-2 A Transition from Hemorrhagic to Artherothrombotic Stroke

As life expectancy increases, acute neurological deficits or strokes may become a significant health problem before there is an increase in coronary heart disease (Reed, 1990). Early in the transition from infectious to noncommunicable diseases, many of the strokes are so-called hemorrhagic strokes, caused by bleeding from an intracerebral artery into the brain. They have a case fatality rate of 80 percent or more (Wolf, 1994). The major risk factor for all forms of stroke is high blood pressure. For hemorrhagic stroke, low blood cholesterol is also a risk factor (Iso et al., 1989; Reed, 1990). As countries develop, their populations may have increased blood pressure before they experience increased blood cholesterol. This would lead to an increase in deaths from hemorrhagic stroke. Later in the transition, stroke mortality may change from the hemorrhagic type to the atherothrombotic type. Atherothrombotic stroke is caused by atherosclerotic plaques in the arteries that supply the brain. These can undergo ulceration or thrombosis, and the pieces of plaque or thrombus that break off may occlude one or more of the arteries to the brain and cause a malfunction. If the blood flow is restored, the malfunction is a transient ischemic attack. If the blood flow is not restored, brain tissue dies as a result of the stroke. This form of stroke has a case fatality rate of approximately 20 percent, but many of the survivors are left with disabilities such as paralysis, inability to speak, or blindness. The risk factors for atherothrombotic strokes are hypertension, elevated blood cholesterol, diabetes, and obesity. Studies of mortality from stroke in rapidly developing country populations have shown consistently high mortality rates and a transition in relative importance from intracerebral hemorrhagic stroke to atherothrombotic stroke with economic development.

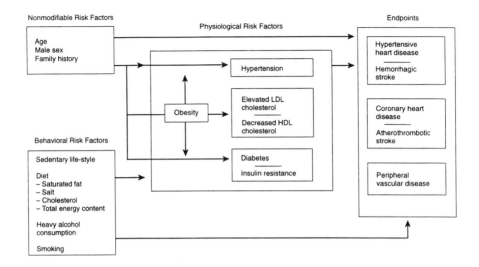

FIGURE 1-2 Relationships among risk factors for cardiovascular disease.

Risk factors that have a causal association with CVD (hypertension, elevated LDL cholesterol, decreased HDL cholesterol, diabetes, cigarette smoking, sedentary life-style) are thought to explain at least 50 percent of the burden of CVD (Pooling Project Research Group, 1978). Interactions among these risk factors can multiply the risk of disease. Additional risk factors have been proposed that help explain the remaining CVD burden. These include the levels of thrombogenic factors such as serum fibrinogen, levels of triglycerides, lipoprotein profiles, levels of serum homocysteine, levels of dietary antioxidants, alcohol consumption, and certain psychosocial factors.

THE GLOBAL BURDEN

Cardiovascular Disease as the Leading Cause of Death

It is likely that CVD became the developing world's leading cause of death for the first time in the mid-1990s. (Murray and Lopez, 1997c)

The Global Burden of Disease Study has estimated the distribution of deaths by region for 1990 (Murray and Lopez, 1997c). Noncommunicable diseases (NCDs) rank first in most developing countries, in developed countries, and worldwide. Moreover, CVD usually accounts for about half of all NCD deaths. The 10 major causes of death in developed and developing countries are listed in Table 1-2. In developing countries, CVD was responsible for slightly fewer deaths than infectious and parasitic diseases in 1990. It is estimated that since that time—with the decreasing incidence of infectious and parasitic diseases and the increasing incidence of CVD in the mid-1990s—CVD became the developing world's leading cause of death. Even in 1990, CVDs were the leading cause of death for all major geographic regions of the developing world except India and Sub-Saharan Africa.

Although CVD mortality is well known to be high for men and for older age groups, it is also the major cause of mortality in the economically productive age group of 30–69 years and in women (Table 1-3). Not surprisingly, in 1990 CVD caused three times as many deaths in 30- to 69-year-old men and women as did infectious and parasitic diseases worldwide. This is true for all regions of the world, except Sub-Saharan Africa, where the number of deaths from CVD and infectious or parasitic diseases was about equal. Recent data suggest that mortality from stroke in Sub-Saharan Africa is higher than previously reported and confirm the relatively young age of the victims (United Republic of Tanzania, 1997).

BOX 1-3 Hypertension: A Global Disease

Elevated blood pressure or hypertension emerges as a major cause of hemorrhagic stroke, hypertensive heart disease, and hypertensive kidney failure even before coronary heart disease and atherothrombotic stroke become major causes of mortality (Whelton et al., 1995). Using a conservative definition for hypertension as blood pressure above 160 mm Hg systolic or above 95 mm Hg diastolic, the prevalence of hypertension, even in Sub-Saharan Africa, ranges from 10 to 33 percent in 30- to 49-year-old men and women (Nissinen et al., 1988). The INTERSALT study carried out in 32 countries, many of them developing, used carefully standardized measurements of blood pressure to confirm substantial prevalence of blood pressures above 140/90 mm Hg in most countries, both developed and developing (INTERSALT Cooperative Research Group, 1988). In addition, the level of awareness worldwide is low, as are treatment and control of elevated blood pressure (Marques-Vidal and Tuomilehto, 1997).

A practical approach to CVD control is primordial prevention (i.e., prevention of the risk factors themselves). Hypertension may be considered either a risk factor for CVD or a disease in itself. This raises the issue of whether hypertension is preventable. Some of its risk factors such as age, male sex, and family history are nonmodifiable. The modifiable risk factors include obesity, sedentary life-style, high-sodium diet, alcohol consumption, and possibly other dietary factors. Clinical trials to prevent the development of hypertension suggest that weight control, increased physical activity, and lower dietary intakes of sodium and alcohol show good potential for primordial prevention (Cutler, 1993). Despite their low cost relative to treatment, these strategies have not yet been investigated in developing countries. Without successful primordial or primary prevention, significant disability and mortality are likely to be caused by hypertension.

Another Measure of Disease Burden

Until recently, quantifying the burden of disease and injury in human populations relied primarily on measurements of mortality. However, using mortality measurements alone ignores significant, nonfatal illness and disability. Because of these and other limitations, different measures for the disease burden have been developed. One of the most commonly used of these is the DALY (disability-adjusted life year), which is a measure of the years of life lost (YLL) due to premature mortality plus years lived with disability (YLD). The years of life lost from premature death are defined as the difference between actual age at death and life expectancy at this age in a low-mortality population. The years of life lived with a disability are adjusted for seven levels of severity of the disability.

When DALYs are used to measure the disease burden, there is a change in the ordering of major diseases or injuries in developing countries (Table 1-4). For developing countries in 1990, CVD ranked fifth as a source of disease burden (measured in DALYs), while it ranked second as a cause of death. Projections for the year 2020 place ischemic heart disease third and cerebrovascular disease fifth among the leading causes of disease burden measured in DALYs for developing countries (Murray and Lopez, 1996). The broader category of CVD would rank even higher than these two subcategories in the global burden of disease and injury. Estimates of the global burden of disease in 2020 can be compared with those for mortality, in which CVD is predicted to be the major contributor in developing as well as developed countries.

TABLE 1-2 The 10 Major Causes of Death in Developed and Developing Countries—1990

Cause of Death	Deaths (thousands)		
	Developed	Developing	World
Cardiovascular disorders	5,245	9,082	14,327
Infectious and parasitic diseases	163	9,166	9,329
Malignant neoplasms	2,413	3,611	6,024
Respiratory infections	389	3,992	4,380
Unintentional injuries	552	2,682	3,233
Respiratory disorders	500	2,435	2,935
Perinatal disorders	82	2,361	2,443
Digestive disorders	424	1,426	1,851
Intentional injuries	282	1,569	1,851
Genitourinary disorders	167	568	735

SOURCE: Murray and Lopez, 1997c.

BOX 1-4 Congestive Heart Failure: The Next Epidemic

Congestive heart failure (CHF) develops as a consequence of disease and dysfunction of the heart. Its signs and symptoms vary, but it generally results in failure of the left heart to provide adequate output. This causes fluid to collect in the lungs and leads to shortness of breath. When the right heart is unable to provide adequate output, there is a buildup of fluid in the body (edema, liver enlargement, etc.). Any disease affecting the heart muscle or valves can lead to heart failure. In Africa and South America, heart failure is likely to be caused by rheumatic valvular disease, whereas in Asia it is likely to be caused by hypertensive heart disease and, in North America and Western Europe, by coronary artery disease. Prevalence estimates from U.S. and European studies suggest that 6 to 10 percent of the elderly population meets criteria for CHF, which increases sharply with age (Cowie et al., 1997). Around 1970, 250,000 new cases of heart failure were diagnosed each year in the United States. In 1988, 400,000 new cases—and in 1992, 700,000 new cases—of CHF were diagnosed, per year (Abraham and Bristow, 1997). CHF now affects 5 million Americans, is the most common cause of hospitalization in persons 65 years and older, and accounts for $10 billion to 40 billion in health care costs. The majority of CHF cases are due to coronary artery disease or hypertensive heart disease. Developing countries could avoid the escalating health care costs currently experienced by developed countries if they could control these diseases.

TABLE 1-3 Deaths (thousands) Due to Cardiovascular Disease and to Infectious and Parasitic Diseases (IPDs) in 30- to 69-Year-Olds by Sex and Region—1990

Region	Men		Women	
	CVD	IPD	CVD	IPD
Established market economies	483	42	227	12
Formerly socialist economies	263	20	163	6
India	611	429	481	240
China	576	158	439	89
Other Asian and Pacific Island countries	289	147	226	140
Sub-Saharan Africa	183	215	211	228
Latin American and Caribbean countries	186	62	147	48
Middle Eastern Crescent	285	83	215	85
Worldwide	3,028	1,128	2,201	798

SOURCE: Murray and Lopez, 1996.

Regional Differences

Populations worldwide have very different levels and presentations of CVD as well as infectious and parasitic diseases. Three factors are likely to contribute to regional differences in CVD:

1. the stage of economic development, which has a role in the predominance of different CVDs,
2. differences in behavior and life-style that expose populations to different levels of risk, and
3. differences in racial and ethnic heritage, which determine genetic predisposition to CVD.

The first factor contributing to regional differences in CVD is the stage of development, as illustrated in Table 1-5. China and India have considerable mortality from rheumatic and inflammatory heart diseases. Sub-Saharan Africa continues to have more mortality from cerebrovascular disease than from ischemic heart disease. These differences are consistent with the level of development of these regions.

The second factor contributing to regional differences in CVD involves the behaviors and life-styles that expose populations to increased levels of risk. The World Health Organization (WHO) Inter-Health Program has documented striking differences in the prevalence of cigarette smoking, hypertension, hypercholesterolemia, and obesity (Berrios et al., 1997; Vartiainen et al., 1991). These differences may determine whether the major CVD is coronary, cerebrovascular, or another presentation. Whereas individuals in developing country populations tend to have a single important risk factor, those in European and North American populations have two or more important risk factors (see Figure 1-3) (Berrios et al., 1997). Since risks for CVD tend to be multiplicative in effect, the greater number of risk factors in developed countries may explain their higher risks.

The third factor contributing to regional differences in CVD is racial and ethnic heritage, which determines the genetic predisposition to CVD. For example, South Asians who migrate to Europe, North America, or other regions of the world have an incidence of CVD that exceeds even the incidence of the countries to which they have migrated (Enas and Mehta, 1995). This suggests a gene–environment interaction (the so-called thrifty gene) in which high caloric intake, a sedentary life-style, or obesity elicits an exaggerated insulin response, that leads to hyperinsulinemia, diabetes, and other physiologic risk factors (McKeige et al., 1993; Neel, 1962). A variation of this observation may be the strikingly low HDL levels and high serum triglyceride levels observed in the Turkish population (Mahley et al., 1995).

TABLE 1-4 Percentage of Disability-Adjusted Life Years Attributable to Specific Causes of Death for Developed and Developing Regions of the World—1990

Disease or Injury	Percentage of Total DALYS		
	Developed	Developing	World
Infectious and parasitic diseases	2.7	25.6	22.9
Neuropsychiatric disorders	22.0	9.0	10.5
Unintentional injuries	10.3	11.1	11.0
Cardiovascular diseases	20.4	8.3	9.7
Respiratory infections	1.6	9.4	8.5
Perinatal disorders	1.9	7.3	6.7
Malignant neoplasms	13.7	4.0	5.1
Respiratory disorders	4.8	4.3	4.4
Intentional injuries	4.2	4.1	4.1
Nutritional deficiencies	0.9	4.1	3.7

SOURCE: Murray and Lopez, 1997c.

TABLE 1-5 Deaths Due to Specific Cardiovascular Diseases for Regions at Different Stages of Development—1990

Region	CVD Deaths (thousands)			
	Rheumatic	Inflammatory	Cerebrovascular	Other
Established market economies	20	65	788	633
Formerly socialist economies	25	39	639	341
India	70	83	448	490
China	163	66	1,272	305
Other Asian and Pacific Island countries	10	82	390	406
Sub-Saharan Africa	20	63	383	140
Latin America and Caribbean countries	8	25	249	160
Middle Eastern Crescent	24	72	212	377

SOURCE: Murray and Lopez, 1997c.

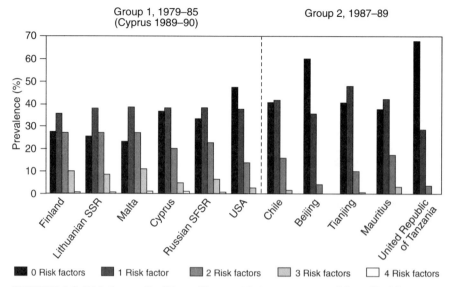

FIGURE 1-3 Risk factors for 35- to 64-year-olds in two groups of Inter-Health countries (data on cholesterol levels and body mass index were not available for Beijing). SOURCE: World Health Organization, 1991. Reprinted with permission.

Barker and Osmond (1992) have proposed that the adult risk for CVD can be determined to a substantial degree by factors in fetal or neonatal life that "program" metabolic regulation for the early dietary environment and do not appear to adapt to the dietary environment of later life. This would explain why low birthweight or relatively low weight gain in the first year appears to predispose a person to later high risk of CVD. This risk factor overrides the positive results that could be expected from interventions in later life. There is some empirical support for this idea, but it requires further investigation. If this programming is confirmed, it provides yet another reason for improving maternal and infant nutrition and health.

Attributable Risk

What proportion of CVD can be attributed to specific risk factors and thus be prevented if these risk factors are controlled? This is a function of the prevalence of a risk factor and of its relative contribution to CVD. A single risk factor can explain a large proportion of the disease, as in the case of African-American women for whom more than 50 percent of total mortality is attributable to hypertension, which is highly prevalent and contributes a large part of the risk for CVD (Deubner et al., 1975). Control of such risk factors has potential for realizing a sizable reduction in the CVD burden.

CONCLUSIONS

CVD has been the dominant cause of death in developed countries for more than half a century. CVD has also emerged as a dominant disease in developing countries, although this is likely to be only the beginning of an epidemic that will continue to emerge. These diseases already affect large numbers of middle-aged persons, both men and women, and all economic groups. They cause three times as many deaths in 39- to 69-year-olds worldwide as do infectious and parasitic diseases combined. Control of CVD requires an understanding of the changing pattern of disease as a region develops and a focus on the risk factors that have so dramatically influenced CVD in the developed world. Where limited data are available in developing countries, as for atherosclerotic disease, the rich databases of developed countries can provide a strong starting point for addressing important risk factors.

2

◆ ◆ ◆ ◆ ◆

The Future Burden of Cardiovascular Diseases in Developing Countries

Cardiovascular disease (CVD) is currently a substantial cause of death and disability in many low- and middle-income countries, and this burden will be higher in the future. Three factors will determine the increase in death and disability from this disease. First, as populations age, more people will reach ages at which CVD becomes common. Second, older populations will be more exposed to risk factors including tobacco, high blood pressure, diets high in saturated fat, obesity, and a sedentary life-style. Third, populations may change their use of preventive and curative health services.

Aging populations are the result of declining fertility and declining mortality in earlier years. The probability of death before age 5 is expected to decrease by half in demographically developing countries—from 11 percent in 1990 to 5 percent in 2020—for both males and females. The probability of death between ages 15 and 60 is expected to decline from 20 to 12 percent for women and to remain close to 24 percent for men over the same period. Estimates suggest that the proportion of adults (both young and older) will rise sharply. Developing countries will have a 108 percent increase in the number of adults aged 30–69 from 1990 to 2020 (Murray and Lopez, 1996; UN, 1995). The number of deaths before age 30 is expected to decline by 41 percent between 1990 and 2020. In contrast, the numbers of deaths between ages 30 and 69 and at age 70 and above are expected to increase by 149 percent and 53 percent, respectively.

PROJECTIONS OF THE FUTURE BURDEN

Projections of the future burden of CVD rely on models because there are few prospective studies in developing countries. Some projections are based solely on current demographic trends (Bulatao and Stephens, 1992), whereas

24

others rely on extrapolation of past trends and population projections. Aging of the population is the only predictive variable in projection models. Murray and Lopez (1996) had the most comprehensive projections for the years 1990 to 2020, and these include estimates for different causes of mortality. The projections rely on an econometric model that has four variables: (1) per capita income, (2) human capital (average number of years of schooling in a population), (3) smoking intensity, and (4) time. They have three levels for future growth— baseline, optimistic, and pessimistic—based on standard, higher, and lower growths in per capita income. The model is applied to each disease and injury group by age group and by sex.

Table 2-1 summarizes the results for CVD using this model for the years 1990 and 2020. Most of the increase in total CVD deaths is due to ischemic heart disease and cerebrovascular disease. The ratio of CVD deaths to total deaths is stable across the baseline (34 percent), optimistic (36 percent), and pessimistic (31 percent) scenarios. In contrast, the contribution of all communicable diseases will differ greatly between baseline (18 percent) and pessimistic (25 percent) scenarios. This reflects the fact that income growth has large impacts on early, but not middle-age, mortality (World Bank, 1993). In rank order of disability-adjusted life years (DALYs), ischemic heart disease and cerebrovascular disease, respectively, will change from being the eighth and tenth largest contributors of disease burden in 1990, to the third and fifth largest contributors in 2020 (Murray and Lopez, 1996).

The increase in CVD mortality projected in Table 2-1 is likely to be conservative. First, the model does not take into account the possible interaction of increases in key risk factors such as tobacco, hypertension, and saturated fat intake. Data from a study of U.S. males suggest that the combination of these three risk factors elevates risk severalfold compared with any single risk factor. Second, the model does not consider the 20 percent increased risk of CVD caused by childhood deprivation, as measured by low birthweight or poor nutritional status (Rich-Edwards et al., 1997). Low birthweight (defined as less than 2,500 grams) is more common in low-income countries, where it averages 16 percent, than in high-income countries, where it averages 6 percent. The highest levels of low birthweight are in South Asia and Sub-Saharan Africa (33 and 16 percent, respectively).

When considering projections for the global burden of CVD, recent trends in the United States show that the long-standing decline in stroke mortality has stopped or even reversed and the decline in mortality from coronary heart disease appears to have stopped. There are also persistent or growing disparities in CVD mortality between white and minority populations, with minority populations at greater risk (AHA, 1998; Labarthe, 1998). Thus, the challenges of controlling CVD continue in the developed countries. There is much yet to be learned through application of R&D to the CVD epidemic in developing countries.

26

TABLE 2-1 Deaths from Cardiovascular Diseases in 1990 and 2020, by Region (thousands)

Region	Cause	Sex	Deaths at All Ages		Percentage of Deaths at All Ages		Deaths at Age 30–69		Percentage of Deaths at Age 30–69	
			1990	2020	1990	2020	1990	2020	1990	2020
Developing country	Ischemic heart disease	Males	1,828	4,347	9	14	899	2,355	12	14
		Females	1,737	3,501	9	15	651	947	12	12
	Cerebrovascular disease	Males	1,461	3,218	7	10	679	1,696	9	10
		Females	1,492	2,775	8	12	582	782	11	10
	Inflammatory and rheumatic heart disease	Males	319	591	2	2	149	370	2	2
		Females	368	448	2	2	162	199	3	2
World	Ischemic heart disease	Males	3,126	6,077	12	16	1,427	3,014	15	16
		Females	3,134	5,030	13	17	904	1,080	14	12
	Cerebrovascular disease	Males	2,022	3,977	8	10	862	1,927	9	10
		Females	2,359	3,721	10	13	729	867	11	10
	Inflammatory and rheumatic heart disease	Males	388	677	2	2	222	414	2	2
		Females	448	544	2	2	192	214	3	2

SOURCE: Murray and Lopez, 1996.

Future Impact of Tobacco

Age-specific mortality and morbidity rates will increasingly be determined by current and future exposure to risks such as tobacco. The relative lack of large, standardized, prospective epidemiologic data in most developing populations makes it difficult to predict trends in tobacco use, high blood pressure, high-fat diets, and obesity. There is enough evidence, however, to suggest that these risks are increasing in many low- and middle-income countries (WHO, 1997).

Currently, only the impact of tobacco can be predicted with some confidence. The contribution of tobacco to the global burden of disease is predicted to increase to about 8.3 million deaths and 124 million DALYs by 2020, with more than 70 percent of these occurring in developing countries. This amounts to a doubling of the percentage of current deaths and a tripling of current DALYs due to tobacco use worldwide (Ad Hoc Committee, 1996). Peto and colleagues (1994) estimated that there will be 10 million tobacco-related deaths annually by 2030—or a total of 100 million deaths over the next 20 years—with half of these occurring in the productive years of middle age (35–69) and causing a 20- to 25-year loss in life expectancy for smokers. These projections are limited by the uncertainty of the impact of past and current smoking patterns. Although current trends predict with some assurance that deaths due to tobacco use will reach 10 million per year, the more difficult prediction is *when* this will happen.

Tobacco has the highest impact in populations with high underlying cardiovascular mortality. South Asian males, for example, have high (and largely unexplained) levels of CVD. Thus, in India, tobacco-attributable mortality is expected to increase from 1 percent of total mortality in 1990 to 13 percent in 2020. Similarly, in males in the former socialist economies (FSEs) tobacco-attributable mortality is expected to increase from 14 percent of total mortality in 1990 to 23 percent in 2020 (Ad Hoc Committee, 1996). A study in the United Kingdom suggested that among cigarette smokers aged 30–49 years, 80 percent of myocardial infarctions were caused by their tobacco use, among those aged 50–59 years, the figure was 67 percent, and among those aged 60–79 years, it was 50 percent.

TABLE 2-2 Estimated Number of CVD Deaths (in millions) Worldwide Attributable to Cigarette Smoking and Percentage of Total Estimated Global Deaths—1990, 2000, 2010, and 2020

	1990	2000	2010	2020
CVD deaths attributable to cigarette smoking	0.96	1.40	1.93	2.61
Percentage of total deaths	1.9	2.5	3.2	3.8

SOURCE: Ad Hoc Committee, 1996.

Future Effects of Other CVD Risk Factors

There are few reliable cross-sectional or prospective data on the contribution of most risk factors to CVD in developing countries. Thus, the projection of such risks into the future is not possible. For developing countries in 1990, Murray and Lopez (1996) estimated that hypertension contributed to 3.8 percent of total deaths and 0.9 percent of total DALYs. Alcohol use contributed to 1.6 percent of total deaths and 2.7 percent of total DALYs. Physical inactivity contributed to 2.3 percent of total deaths and 0.6 percent of total DALYs.

Elevated blood pressure is a significant cause of ischemic heart disease and stroke worldwide and may have greater effects in East Asian countries (MacMahon et al., 1990). The determinants of elevated blood pressure appear to be similar for different populations. The INTERSALT study of 52 populations (including 17 in developing countries and 5 in FSEs) revealed that urinary sodium (a proxy for sodium intake), body mass index, and high alcohol intake are correlated with high blood pressure. In Western countries, processed foods are the main source of sodium, which contributes significantly to hypertension (INTERSALT, 1988; Law et al., 1991). Consumption of processed foods is increasing in developing countries (WHO, 1992).

Levels of saturated fat intake and blood cholesterol appear to be rising in FSEs and developing countries. With increasing affluence, the consumption of meat and saturated fat rises, and this trend is likely to occur globally (WHO, 1992), particularly where subsidies are given to meat and dairy producers. In urban China, mean body mass index, blood pressure, and cholesterol rose over a three-year period in the late 1980s (Keil and Kuulasmaa, 1989). A study in rural and urban India found values of body mass index, blood pressure, fasting blood cholesterol, and diabetes approaching those of Indian populations in the West.

Evidence is emerging to suggest that obesity is increasing rapidly in developing as well as developed countries. Moreover, since it appears to be escalating in children as well as adults, the health consequences may continue into the distant future. Reliable data are available for only a few developing countries to show increasing obesity over time. In African and Asian countries, obesity is still relatively uncommon, but more prevalent in urban than rural populations (Mbanya et al., 1997).

Diabetes is another independent risk factor for CVD. Its prevalence in adults worldwide was 4 percent in 1995 and is projected to rise to 35 percent or more by the year 2025 (King et al., forthcoming). Although the prevalence of diabetes is higher in developed than in developing countries, the number of adults with diabetes worldwide will rise from 135 million in 1995 to 300 million in the year 2025. The major part of this increase will occur in developing countries: by the year 2025, more than 75 percent of persons with diabetes will reside in these countries. In absolute terms, the countries having the greatest number of people with diabetes are—and will continue to be in the year 2025—India, China, and the United States. Diabetes is more common in women than men, especially in

Latin America and the Caribbean, China, and developed countries. In India, more men than women have diabetes. Diabetes will become increasingly concentrated in urban areas. In developing countries, the majority of persons with diabetes are 45–64 years of age, whereas in developed countries, they are 65 years and over. This pattern is predicted to persist to the year 2025.

CAN DEVELOPING COUNTRIES AVOID
THE FUTURE BURDEN?

Changes in coronary heart disease mortality in different populations over periods of only a few years demonstrate the strength of environmental determinants of risk regardless of the underlying genetic composition of those populations. The challenge is to address these environmental determinants effectively, even before research identifies specific subgroups with exceptional genetic risk (Breslow, 1997; Labarthe, 1998). Although CVD mortality early in the epidemiologic transition tends to be highest among the well educated and affluent, most countries that have undergone the epidemiologic transition also observe CVD mortality to be high in population groups with low levels of income and education. Epidemiologic studies in upper- and middle-income countries provide strong evidence for the preventability of CVD (Blackburn, 1997; Dowse et al., 1995). This evidence includes differences in CVD incidence among populations; trends in CVD incidence over time; CVD incidence among migrants; trends of CVD incidence with changes in exposure to risk factors; correlations between risk factor exposure and disease in individuals and populations; estimates of risk reduction due to changing distributions of risk factors in populations; results of clinical trials with risk factor modification; and results of public health trials of population-based risk factor modification (Pearson and Stone, 1997). Together these form a strong rationale to support the CVD risk factor paradigm, which states that controlling major CVD risk factors should control the disease itself.

Although death in middle age need not be common in any population, death in old age is unavoidable, and in some cultures, attempts to avoid it are not acceptable. In the 1880s, 50 percent of U.K. residents died before age 40, and 77 percent before age 70. By 1980, only 3 percent of U.K. residents died before age 40, and 30 percent died before age 70. In both periods, nearly all died before age 100. Evidence that CVD can be avoided also comes from the wide divergence of CVD mortality across populations (Thom, 1989), from international and internal migration studies (Reed and MacLean, 1989), and from changes over time. Analyses from Norway suggest that the scarcity of saturated fat, cigarettes, and alcohol during the Second World War contributed to marked declines in certain chronic diseases (Thelle, 1985).

Second, certain middle-income countries in Latin America (Chile, Argentina, Uruguay, and Cuba) have shown a marked decline in CVD mortality. Mauritius showed marked declines in serum cholesterol, hypertension, and smoking from 1987 to 1992 (Dowse, 1995). In Poland there was a one-third decline in mortality due to CVD in men and women aged 20–40 between 1991 and 1993. This appears to be attributable in large part to a declining dietary intake of saturated fats—the ratio of polyunsaturated to saturated fats increased from 0.2 to 0.4 in a short time. Declines in saturated fat intake and increases in vegetable fats are consistent with the end of government subsidies to meat and dairy producers (Zatonski, 1996).

Several FSEs have shown marked increases in CVD mortality rates, but the reasons have not been well studied. In many countries, increases follow recent declines. Underlying reasons appear to be the maturing tobacco epidemic, increased saturated fat intake, elevated blood pressure, and poor access to primary and secondary preventive care. The role of risk factors remains poorly understood but offers opportunities for research. Rising incomes may increase tobacco use, use of processed food with high salt content, diets high in saturated fat, and obesity. These effects depend also on the level of information available. For example, in 1970, tobacco use increased with increasing income for males in developed countries. By 1990, however, tobacco use was decreasing with rising income, due partly to better and more available information on its hazards.

Developed countries have shown a remarkable decline in CVD mortality. Canada, for example, has about 40 percent fewer CVD deaths than predicted by 1970 age-standardized rates (Second International Heart Health Conference, 1995). Most declines appear to be driven by gradual life-style changes, declining tobacco consumption, improved diets, and other less understood factors. The rapid declines in Poland, Estonia, and Norway are due to marked socioeconomic changes. The continuing experience in many FSEs may provide new understanding.

Finally, clinical treatments have contributed to the decline of CVD in developed countries, largely by offering wide access to low-cost medical treatment rather than high-technology clinical or surgical treatment. For example, the improved survival from acute myocardial infarction after 1980 is due largely to increasing use of aspirin, low-cost beta-blockers, and to a lesser extent, newer and more expensive clot-dissolving drugs (Forrester et al., 1996).

Cardiovascular Disease Prevention Strategies

Two strategies might be employed for CVD prevention: one that focuses on high-risk individuals and one that focuses on a public health approach (Figure 2-1) (Carleton et al., 1991). The first approach identifies those with high exposure to CVD risk factors and intensively treats them to reduce that risk. Although it is effective for individuals, this approach has limited impact on the population-wide burden of disease, since most cases are not at high risk. The public health approach is to shift the entire distribution of CVD risk factors to a lower level. In reality, many populations use a combination of the two strategies.

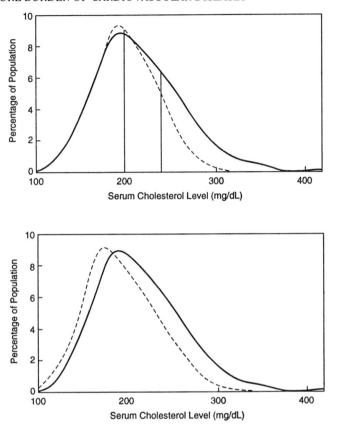

FIGURE 2-1 Cholesterol distribution in the U.S. population aged 20–74 years from the National Health and Nutrition Examination Survey II (1976–1980) and potential changes in this distribution. **Top:** Expected shift in population distribution of serum cholesterol values with application of high-risk approach (Adult Treatment Panel Guidelines of National Cholesterol Education Program). Dashed line shows effect of the recommendations. **Bottom:** Expected shift in population distribution of serum cholesterol values with application of public health approach (Population Panel of the National Cholesterol Education Program). Dashed line shows effect of the recommendations. SOURCE: Carleton et al., 1991. Copyright 1991 by the American Heart Association; reprinted with permission.

Efficacy of Current Interventions

The remarkable reduction in CVD mortality documented in the populations of Western Europe, North America, Australia, and New Zealand since 1970 suggests that population-wide efforts are effective in lowering the disease burden. More controlled studies of interventions in schools, work sites, and entire communities have had less certain results but are successful when the intervention is more intense (Pearson and Stone, 1997).

Primary prevention of CVD has been effective in randomized trials that lower CVD risks such as elevated low-density lipoprotein (LDL) cholesterol, high-fat or high-cholesterol diets, hypertension, and cigarette smoking (Forrester et al., 1996; Pasternak et al., 1996). The efficacy of these interventions in the United States has lead to the development of guidelines (Grundy et al., 1997). In general, persons at low risk are encouraged to develop healthier life-styles, and pharmacologic therapies are reserved for high-risk individuals. Primary preventive interventions can be relatively cost-effective, especially for low-cost interventions and subgroups of the population at high risk (Goldman et al., 1996).

Case management strategies have been investigated extensively for patients with both acute and chronic manifestations of coronary heart disease and cerebrovascular disease. Interventions range from relatively inexpensive steps such as the control of high-risk behavior (e.g., smoking cessation, lipid-lowering diet, physical activity, weight reduction) to the use of inexpensive technologies (e.g., lipid-lowering drugs, aspirin, beta-blockers, estrogens) to sophisticated, expensive technologies (e.g., thrombolytic therapies, automated internal defibrillation, coronary angiography with or without angioplasty and/or stent placement, coronary bypass surgery, cardiac transplantation). Guidelines for the management of acute myocardial infarction (Ryan et al., 1996) and secondary prevention strategies (Smith et al., 1995) have been published for the United States. In case management, behavioral changes and inexpensive technologies are highly cost-effective (Goldman et al., 1996).

Although little information is available from developing countries about the feasibility and cost-effectiveness of such management strategies, the committee believes that increasing the use of one or several effective, low-cost medications (aspirin and/or beta-blockers) in survivors of acute myocardial infarction could dramatically reduce CVD deaths in developing countries. As indicated in Table 2-3, the relatively low-cost combination of aspirin and beta-blockers after acute myocardial infarction could avoid about 300,000 deaths due to ischemic heart disease (IHD) and stroke in low- and middle-income countries in the year 2020, if coverage is increased from 30–40 percent to 85 percent of the patient population.[*] If more people with acute myocardial infarction are treated and if the use

---

[*]This analysis assumes that (1) the number of cases will be 2.5 times that of estimated deaths; (2) half of the cases access care (the remainder die or are untreated); (3) in-hospital mortality is 10 percent for ages 30–45, 15 percent for ages 45–60, 20 percent for ages 60–69, and 25 percent for ages 70 and over; (4) the current use of aspirin or beta-blockers is 20–40 percent in men and 10 percent lower in women; and (5) the relative reduction in risk of death is 25 percent.

of aspirin and beta-blockers is equally high, it is estimated that 400,000 deaths could be avoided in developing countries.

It has been shown in developed countries that when survivors of myocardial infarction stop smoking, there is a profound reduction of mortality. Research on ways to promote smoking cessation deserves support.

ECONOMIC CONSEQUENCES

The economic consequences of the increasing CVD burden include household health and composition, lost production and earnings, and lost investment and consumption (Over et al., 1994). Few studies exist in developing or developed countries to document these economic losses.

The death of an adult family member can have a devastating impact on the household. In Bangladesh, the probability of death between ages 15 and 60 is 29 percent for females and 31 percent for males. When there is an adult death—most often from CVD—a child of less than 2 years has a 12-fold higher probability of death (Over et al., 1994).

In developing country populations, CVD occurs at an earlier age than in developed country populations. There is a greater loss of productivity and a greater impact on the household. In India, mortality, years of life lost discounted at 3 percent, and productivity-weighted years of life lost (YLL) (productivity weight maximal at age 24) show different patterns (see Table 2-4). In the productivity-weighted years of life lost the greatest loss is during the productive years of middle age.

Data from the United States suggest that reduced productivity and lost output due to CVD cost about $17.6 billion in 1993, or 15 percent of the total economic costs of CVD (including facilities, services, and drugs; AHA, 1993). Total costs for CVD were about 2 percent of the gross domestic product (GDP), while reduced productivity and lost output due to CVD amounted to about 0.3 percent of the GDP. In Canada, CVD accounts for 21 percent of total disease-classifiable costs of illness or a total of U.S. $12 billion per year (HSF, 1994). These costs include treatment, care, and indirect costs, such as the loss of income from mortality and disability. CVD costs are followed by those from injuries (16 percent of the total) and cancer (11 percent). CVD is responsible for the highest proportion (32 percent) of earnings lost due to premature death and is followed by cancer (27 percent); CVD accounts for 17 percent of lost productivity due to disability.

TABLE 2-3 2020: Number and Percentage of Total IHD and Stroke Deaths Avoided by Use of Aspirin, Beta-Blockers, and Increased Treatment

Age	Aspirin and Beta-Blockers (85% use of aspirin and beta-blockers)		Aspirin, Beta-Blockers, and Treatment (10% increase in treatment)	
	Developing Countries	FSEs	Developing Countries	FSEs
30–69	72,000 (2%)	38,000 (3%)	96,000 (3%)	45,000 (3.5%)
All ages	211,000 (2.5%)	102,000 (3.5%)	281,000 (3.5%)	122,000 (4%)

SOURCE: Ad Hoc Committee, 1996.

TABLE 2-4 Estimates of Mortality in India by Age Group Using Different Weighting Scales—1992

Age	Percentage of Deaths	YLL at 3% Discount Rate	Productivity-Weighted YLL
<30	41.6	59.1	29.0
30–69	32.8	29.6	45.0
≥70	25.5	11.3	26.0

NOTE: World Bank estimates of mortality differ from the Global Burden of Disease Study results presented due to the different populations studied.

SOURCE: Jha et al., forthcoming.

As has been noted, developing countries are likely in two to three decades to have a CVD burden comparable to that of developed countries today. However, economic projections suggest that developing countries will not be able to afford expensive cardiovascular procedures and specialists' services (Jha et al., forthcoming). Western-based technologies have increased rapidly in the urban settings of many developing countries, often spurred by inappropriate government incentives.

Control of rising CVD costs will have to rely on the following guidelines: (1) public policies that subsidize prevention and low-cost clinical care ahead of more expensive curative interventions; (2) the use of appropriate technology assessment for new devices; and (3) alignment of health finance and delivery systems to ensure a focus on prevention and low-cost clinical care.

COST-EFFECTIVENESS OF PREVENTION AND TREATMENT

Identifying appropriate public policies for the financing and delivery of cardiovascular care relies partly on analyses of cost-effectiveness. These analyses demonstrate that massive policy-based tobacco control campaigns are cost-effective at U.S. $20–$70 per year of life saved (Jha et al., forthcoming). The cost-effectiveness of treatment, on the other hand, depends largely on the cost and use of medications, given that the effectiveness of most treatments ranges from 20 to 30 percent. Thus, a large impact on the population may be possible only if these drugs are widely accessible and low cost. Aspirin and beta-blockers can be cost-effective in emerging market economies and in many low- and middle-income countries. Cholesterol-lowering statin drugs are expensive in developed countries; thus, their cost-effectiveness is currently unfavorable compared with aspirin or beta-blockers (Goldman et al., 1988). However, such statins are less expensive in developing countries, and most of their patents will expire within 5 years. Thus, there is good reason for introducing them into an essential vascular package. Some middle-income countries might be able to introduce more tertiary services into a cost-effective package. In Mauritius, for example, angioplasty is sufficiently cost-effective to be included in a minimal package of interventions (World Bank, 1997a).

3

♦ ♦ ♦ ♦ ♦

Prevention and Treatment of Cardiovascular Diseases in Developing Countries

Health care spending varies dramatically among countries. For example, in 1992 the United States spent approximately $3,000 per person annually on health care, while the Organization for Economic Cooperation and Development (OECD) average was $1,374 (Ad Hoc Committee, 1996). The funding allocated to prevention compared with treatment also varies among countries; however, these figures are more difficult to obtain. Most governments and private agencies support a mix of prevention and treatment efforts (e.g., educational campaigns to reduce cardiac risk factors and acute care centers that provide state-of-the-art diagnostic equipment and treatment). This chapter addresses current efforts in the prevention and treatment of cardiovascular disease (CVD) in developing countries.

DIFFICULTIES IN ASSESSING PATTERNS

Three problems complicate the assessment of current patterns of prevention and care of CVD. The first is the difficulty analyzing the data available. Government health care budgets, which are the primary source of support for prevention and treatment, are often assigned to ministries or divisions without designating the specific programs to be supported. It is, therefore, difficult to identify the part of the budget allocated to CVD and even more difficult to identify the allocations to prevention and treatment of CVD.

The expenditures for health care by the governments of South Korea and Cameroon provide examples of the allocations being made by middle- and low-income countries. The South Korean health care budget for 1996 was allocated from the Ministry of Health and Social Welfare and comprised 10.5 percent of

37

the government's budget. It has four categories: (1) public health education (approximately U.S. $44 million, or 18 percent); (2) communicable disease control (approximately U.S. $64 million, or 26 percent); (3) chronic and mental disease control (approximately U.S. $75 million, or 30 percent); and (4) medical and pharmaceutical programs (approximately U.S. $62 million, or 25 percent). Funding expended on prevention and treatment of CVD could come from three of the four categories, but no information is available on it (Republic of Korea Ministry of Health and Welfare, 1996, 1997).

Health expenditures in Cameroon for the same year (1996) were three percent of the national budget, and assigned to the Ministry of Health. This funding was divided into three categories: personnel and salaries (55 percent), pharmaceuticals (4 percent), and buildings and equipment (41 percent) (W. Muna, personal communication, November 1997).

The second problem in assessing health care expenditures is the several sources of funding. Although government supports the majority of health care services, other agencies have programs that target CVD prevention and care. These include nonprofit organizations (religious and nonreligious), international agencies, and the private sector. There is currently no compilation of data on programs for CVD prevention and cure for any developing country.

The third problem in assessing health care expenditures is the difficulty of categorizing the data. Although sales data are available for aspirin in specific countries, use of aspirin for CVD prevention and treatment are not separated from other uses. Even CVD uses may be for primary prevention (to minimize risk of myocardial infarction or stroke) or for secondary prevention (to prevent a second myocardial infarction). Secondary prevention of CVD further complicates assessing budget allocations. For example, the cost of treatment for heart failure is more than $70 billion annually in the United States alone. Prescribing angiotensin-converting enzyme (ACE) inhibitors in patients with reduced cardiac function decreases the incidence of heart failure, thereby improving the health status of the individual with documented coronary heart disease and reducing health care costs (SOLVD, 1991). Such secondary prevention can dramatically decrease CVD costs. The pharmaceutical data available in developing countries do not, however, address whether an ACE inhibitor is given to prevent the onset of heart failure symptoms or to treat the symptoms of advanced heart failure.

THE ROLE OF INTERNATIONALLY SPONSORED PROGRAMS

Over the past two decades, several programs developed have been directed toward prevention and control of noncommunicable diseases in general, and many activities targeted CVD risk factors. Five international programs are particularly important for CVD prevention (Grabowsky et al., 1997). Each has a network of collaborating centers or societies linked by shared protocols for demonstration projects:

1. *The Countrywide Integrated Noncommunicable Diseases Intervention (CINDI) Program.* Initiated by the World Health Organization (WHO) in 1984, this program involves 24 member countries, among them Canada and European and East European countries (including Russia and Estonia). Several member countries have developed similar protocols and evaluation methods and conducted national demonstration programs. For example, an antismoking campaign, "Quit and Win," in 13 countries involved approximately 15,000 people. CINDI created a CINDI EuroHealth Action Plan, which will focus on multiple risk reduction through community and primary care programs.

2. *Conjuncto de Acciones para la Reducion Multifactorial de las Enfermedades No Transmisibles (CARMEN).* This program was initiated in 1995 by the Pan American Health Organization to develop cardiac risk factor reduction programs in Latin American and the Caribbean. Participating countries begin with demonstration projects that are based on CINDI protocols and designed to reduce risk factors such as smoking, high blood pressure, obesity, diabetes, and excessive alcohol consumption.

3. *The InterAmerican Heart Foundation.* The overall mission of this foundation, formed in 1994, is to reduce disability and death caused by CVD and stroke in populations in North, Central, and South America and the Caribbean. Cardiac risk factors are targeted, along with risk factors for rheumatic fever and Chagas' disease. The program, supported by the International Society and Federation of Cardiology and the American Heart Association, promotes partnerships between medical and nonmedical groups to influence health policy and provide educational resources for CVD risk factor campaigns for member organizations.

4. *Interhealth.* This is an international, collaborative program established in 1984 by WHO. It has 15 members, about one-third of which are developing countries. Although the purpose is to reduce the risks of all noncommunicable diseases, CVD is a focus. Participants monitor the incidence and change in risk factors and have designed community-based demonstration projects.

5. *The Interhealth Nutrition Initiative.* This program, developed in 1993 by WHO, monitors global trends in food and nutrition intake and evaluates dietary risk factors for CVD and other noncommunicable diseases.

THE ROLE OF THE PRIVATE SECTOR

In calculating the ratio of prevention to care for CVD, R&D expenditures by the private-sector are an important component of both prevention and treatment of CVD. The market for pharmaceuticals and medical devices to treat cardiovascular conditions is a large one. The overall expenditure on pharmaceuticals was $220 billion (or $40 per capita) and on medical devices and equipment about $71 billion in 1992 (Ballance et al., 1992). Although the current budget for cardiovascular-related expenditures is unknown, an increase can be anticipated in line with increasing incidence of CVD (Murray and Lopez, 1996).

The proportion of spending directed to pharmaceuticals is higher in both public and private spending in developing countries than developed countries. For example, in 1992 the public and private sectors together spent 10–30 percent of their health care costs ($44 billion), on pharmaceuticals and equipment in developing countries, compared to approximately 5–20 percent of health care budgets in developed countries (IOM, 1997).

Just as health care expenditures do not necessarily translate to improved health status as measured by life expectancy (World Bank, 1993), the proportion of spending for prevention versus treatment may not translate to improved health status. However, most research supports the efficacy of allocating resources to prevention over treatment (Azar and Hofman, 1995; Brownson et al., 1995; King et al., 1995; Krumholz et al., 1993). The applicability of these findings to CVD in developing countries remains to be established.

ZAMBIA: A CASE STUDY

Zambia is a relatively large country with an area of almost 753,000 km^2. The population of 8 million is widely scattered across the country, with 45 percent in rural areas and 55 percent in urban areas. Health care is provided by government institutions, religious organizations, industries (particularly mining companies), the armed services, and practitioners and traditional healers in the private sector. Of these, the government has been the principal provider of care through hospitals and health centers. Religious orders are the second source of care, providing approximately 30 percent of all hospital beds (Martin, 1994).

After independence in 1964, the government made a commitment to increase health care for rural populations—a segment that had received little attention prior to this time. Much of this commitment involved increasing hospital beds. Between 1964 and 1987, the number of hospital beds increased from 10,800 to 22,800. These early efforts to improve health care were aimed at treatment rather than prevention, and particularly the treatment of communicable diseases. Moreover, the pattern of allocation of government budgets consistently favored large urban hospitals. For example, in 1980, 3 percent of the population in one urban area received 60 percent of the national health expenditure. The focus on expanding hospital beds meant that Zambia had one of the highest ratios of hospital beds to population in Sub-Saharan Africa (Martin, 1994).

A severe economic decline began in 1975, which led Zambia to becoming one of six countries in 1991 to lose its status as a middle-income country. With the economic decline of the late 1970s, the government was unable to maintain its commitment to strengthen the health infrastructure by increasing hospital beds. In 1980, primary health care was introduced by the national government with implementation at the district level to encourage community participation.

The government provided the health care workers with training focused on prevention. This change responded to a range of serious but preventable health problems and to correct the previous emphasis on treatment and infrastructure. These efforts were rewarded by an increase in female life expectancy from 45 to 57.5 years and in male life expectancy from 41.8 to 55.4 years over the 28-year period between 1964 and 1992 (Lowther and Moonde, 1994).

This experience in Zambia illustrates the issues involved in setting priorities for CVD. The improved life expectancy and high immunization coverage of Zambians has created longer life expectancy, and a population needing assistance with CVD prevention. As for many countries, the health care expenditures focus on treatment and hospital infrastructure rather than prevention. A preliminary review of 30 developing countries reveals that at least half of total recurrent public health spending supports hospitals (Barnum and Kutzin, 1993). The demands on governments worldwide for inappropriate curative services may be due, in part, to a lack of information about what is cost-effective. The emphasis on treatment over prevention results in health care systems being oriented to expensive technologies for diagnosis and treatment of heart disease, rather than to community and medical education programs to reduce the risk of CVD. Transferring the Western paradigm of health care will place unrealistic burdens on health care systems with extremely limited resources.

FUTURE DIRECTIONS

In summary, few data are available on budget allocations by governments to CVD prevention and treatment. The importance of emphasizing the prevention of CVD and its sequelae is recognized by governments and health authorities of some developing countries and is reflected in their prevention and treatment protocols. However, these countries are in the minority. Most have not recognized the increasing role of CVD in disease burden or have recognized it and chosen to dedicate important resources to building and supporting acute care facilities for the diagnosis and treatment of CVD in urban centers.

Systematic research is needed to answer the following questions: In developing countries, what is the ratio of money allocated to the prevention of CVD compared to its treatment? Does this ratio have an impact on health status as measured by life expectancy or on the distribution of cardiovascular health within populations? What is the cost-effectiveness of secondary prevention efforts? How does a country develop an optimal combination of governmental and private-sector support for effective prevention and treatment of CVD? What is the role of the public and private sectors in preventing CVD? Can developing country governments work with the private sector to reduce the burden of CVD, or is the private sector engaged only in treatment? These questions await appropriate exploration.

4

♦ ♦ ♦ ♦ ♦

Current Research and Development in Developing Countries

Cardiovascular disease (CVD) research in developed countries has built a scientific base for defining disease risk and recognizing when to intervene. It has also provided a rationale for changing personal behaviors that increase the risk for CVD and for developing public health policy and programs. The scientific base can be transferred to developing countries, along with the experience of building R&D capacity. Establishing R&D capacity involves capacity building, technical assistance, and grants for research studies. Capacity building creates the trained human resources and appropriate technical approaches to assess the health needs of the developing country population. Technical assistance provides the experiential base to plan, conduct, and analyze research projects. Research grants can support the cost of conducting research projects.

The committee sought information on the levels and types of R&D currently supporting CVD prevention and treatment in developing countries. Since there are no published data on organizational funding flows, a questionnaire was sent to 26 international donors. Fifteen funders responded to the four questions, and their responses are summarized below:

Question 1: *What is the total annual amount that your organization has spent for the past 10 years on the prevention and treatment of CVD in developing countries?*

Only three organizations indicated supporting such programs during 1987–1996. Reported funding in 1996 U.S. dollars was approximately $635,000, $236,000, and $42,000. The other respondents indicated that they had no programs supporting CVD prevention and treatment in developing countries.

Question 2: *What is the total annual amount that your organization has spent for the past 10 years on research and development in support of total disease prevention and treatment in developing countries?*

Four organizations responded to this question. Their respective spending on R&D for total disease prevention and treatment in developing countries over the past 10 years amounted to approximately U.S. $4.8 million, $83 million, $123 million, and $2 million.

Question 3: *What is the total annual amount that your organization has spent for the past 10 years on research and development in support of CVD prevention and treatment in developing countries?*

One of the 15 respondents reported CVD research funding was approximately U.S. $42,000.

Question 4: *In view of the emerging epidemic of CVD in developing countries, what is the total amount your organization proposes to spend annually over the next 10 years on R&D in support of CVD prevention and treatment in developing countries?*

None of the responses indicated that a commitment had been made at the time to research support for CVD.

Although results of this survey can capture information about grant or contract support, indirect support of capacity building (training on-site or in the donor country or technical assistance provided by donor country professionals) may not be captured.

In summary, relatively little grant or contract funding is currently directed toward the support of CVD prevention and treatment in developing countries, and of this very little supports R&D.

5

♦ ♦ ♦ ♦ ♦

Priorities for Global Research and Development

CONTEXT

As developing countries undergo the epidemiologic transition, cardiovascular disease (CVD) epidemics are emerging or accelerating (Murray and Lopez, 1997a; Reddy and Yusuf, 1998; WHO, 1996, 1997). Depending on the level of development, the pace of the transition varies, although the general process and direction is similar for all countries. The challenge of the epidemiologic transition, therefore, is not whether it will happen in developing countries, but whether it is possible to traverse quickly from the early stage of nutritional and infectious disorders that affect the young to the later stage of noncommunicable diseases (NCDs) that affect mainly the elderly, thus averting or abbreviating the midstage of NCD epidemics when there is a major impact on individuals in their productive middle years. Knowledge of CVD and other NCDs, gained from research conducted primarily in developed countries, can help speed the transition. Local research is required, however, to adapt current knowledge to specific developing country situations.

Policies related to CVD control, as well as priorities for research, must address the emerging epidemic from a long-term perspective. Increases in CVD risk factors precede the CVD epidemic so that strategies for CVD control must focus on the prevention of risk factors as well as their reduction. Control of risk factors may involve: prevention of risk factor development or progression in communities and age groups currently at low risk (primordial prevention); recognition and reduction of high risk in populations that have already acquired an adverse risk profile (primary prevention); and risk factor modification to minimize further complications in those who have clinical disease (secondary prevention). In addition, cost-effective clinical care is needed to improve both the

44

survival and the quality of life of persons who have developed CVD. Appropriately focused research will be necessary to meet each of these goals.

This chapter discusses key areas of research for effective CVD prevention and control in developing countries. Recommendations are presented in bold type both here and in the Executive Summary.

RESEARCH PRIORITIES

There are four criteria to be used in setting priorities for investing in CVD R&D in developing countries:

1. Investments should have a large-scale impact on populations that include men and women, all socioeconomic groups, and various regions of a country. Incremental implementation may be necessary in many countries.

2. Investments in a country should involve methods and processes (but not necessarily results) that are broadly transferable to other low- and middle-income countries.

3. Investments should yield results within a time frame of 5–10 years, although evaluation may be desirable over a longer term.

4. Investments should focus on measurable data that use, for the most part, established epidemiologic, health policy, economic, and social behavioral methodologies.

The main categories of research activity and key recommendations within these categories follow.

Improve Knowledge of the Size of the CVD Burden in Developing Countries

Vital Registration

A sample registration system collects vital statistics on a sample of the population in each state. Such systems are incomplete or nonexistent for many developing countries. About 18 percent of global CVD mortality occurs in China, where the sample registration covers only about 10 percent of the population or about 100 million people in rural and urban settings. About 17 percent of global CVD mortality occurs in India, which has no complete registration system. Registration of vital statistics and cause of death is generally lacking for Africa, Middle Eastern countries, and Asian islands (Murray and Lopez, 1997b).

There are several options for vital registration, the key for each being complete coverage of all deaths, including those from CVD, classified at least by age and sex. Priority assistance should be given to countries that currently lack vital registration systems. Appropriate sampling frames should be built into each system to allow identification of geographic, ethnic, and rural and urban differences in CVD mortality and morbidity.

In developing countries, most vital registries are government funded and lack a research component. These need to develop improved methods for vital registration. In countries with inadequate registration systems, this may include consideration of the capture–recapture method for deriving better estimates of total deaths.

Cause-of-Death Statistics

These provide information on the underlying reasons for death. They are available for developed countries and, to a lesser extent, for Latin America. In China, cause-of-death data are derived from a systematic follow-up of one million deaths to determine their causes and from the district surveillance points system (DSP), which includes about 145 communities in urban and rural settings. In India, cause-of-death data are collected through verbal autopsies on 0.5 percent of rural deaths (Murray and Lopez, 1997b). Both the Chinese and the Indian systems suffer from methodological problems. In China, death rates may be underreported by as much as 30 percent, although unofficial estimates of 8 percent in urban areas and 15 percent in rural areas have been suggested (unpublished data). The Indian system has up to 25 percent of deaths classified as senile or ill-defined. These deaths are likely to include ischemic heart disease, stroke, or other CVD deaths, which would lead to an underestimation of CVD mortality.

Ascertaining cause-specific mortality could be strengthened through the use of community-based random samples, sentinel sites, and surveillance systems modeled after those used in the MONICA study, as well as verbal autopsy techniques to determine the cause of death of adults (especially CVD-related deaths). Data from Tanzania suggest that most deaths occur at home (United Republic of Tanzania, 1997), so including these will require a special effort.

Establishing and evaluating sentinel registration sites, along with validating and using verbal autopsy techniques, are also priority areas for research support.

There is a need to assess the utility of cause-of-death statistics available through the extensive missionary health care network throughout Asia and Africa. Umbrella organizations, such as the Christian Medical and Dental Society, which has more than 400 physician members, have expressed interest in cooperating in this effort. Church groups account for 36 percent of health care in Kenya and more than 50 percent in Cameroon.

Disability Estimates

Most developing countries lack culturally relevant estimates of disability due to CVD and other causes. Estimates of morbidity are not standardized across populations. Focused pilot studies could generate such estimates through validation of a standard quality-of-life measure.

To improve knowledge of the size of the CVD burden in developing countries, the committee recommends the following:

• creating standardized surveys using networks such as the MONICA model (including selected sentinel sites) to monitor cardiovascular mortality levels and trends of clinical events, and the CINDI and CARMEN models to monitor cardiovascular risk factors;
• expanding national and regional systems for vital registration;
• improving the accuracy and completeness of cause-of-death statistics; and
• developing better estimates of disability.

Establishing the Levels, Determinants, and Consequences of Risk Factors

Cross-Sectional Surveys

A major goal of cross-sectional surveys of risk factors is to describe the prevalence and distribution of risk factors, by age, sex, and ethnicity, in representative samples of the population. Such studies of CVD would require moderately large sample sizes (several tens of thousands or hundreds of thousands) and focused, simple data collection. Like vital registration, cross-sectional surveys require a valid sampling frame. Ideally, the data from local cross-sectional studies can be linked to local estimates of the magnitude of various risk factors that are drawn from case-control or prospective studies. Survey data can also be linked to local mortality data.

Cross-sectional surveys are repeated at regular intervals to assess trends in the levels and distribution of risk factors. These surveys could also quantify the association of a CVD risk factor with disease. For this purpose the surveys would be designed to repeat observations of many individuals and to take independent samples during successive surveys. Follow-up of patients in many developing country populations is difficult due to the lack of vital registration systems, the mobility of the population, and variable access to medical care. In these populations it may be easier to classify mortality status than to record nonfatal CVD events. Cross-sectional studies of CVD would have to be sufficiently large to permit follow-up for mortality outcomes.

Analytic Studies

Retrospective case-control or prospective studies can provide estimates of the magnitude of disease risk associated with various CVD risk factors. Such studies should focus on major conditions such as myocardial infarction and on established risk factors such as tobacco use, high blood pressure, high serum cholesterol, diabetes-related syndromes, physical inactivity, and obesity. There is also a need for biochemical studies of risk factors such as apolipoproteins, fibrinogen and other clotting factors, albumin, homocysteine, folate, dietary antioxidants, and infectious agents such as *Chlamydia*, *Helicobacter*, and cytomegalovirus. Such studies, conducted selectively, could confirm the role of CVD and its risk factors in previously underinvestigated populations.

• **Case-control studies of the incidence of disease** can identify the strength of association of a risk factor with CVD and may also uncover new risk factors. Although prospective studies are more robust methodologically because exposure to a risk factor demonstrably precedes disease, retrospective case-control studies can usually generate needed data more quickly and at lower cost. Ideally, cases of disease incidence (e.g., initial myocardial infarction) should be studied to avoid biases in the recording of risk factors. Key conditions for study by case-control methods are acute myocardial infarction, acute stroke, transient ischemic attacks, congestive heart failure, and peripheral vascular disease.

• **Prospective studies** have the advantage of measuring exposure to a risk factor prior to the development of disease. By necessity, these studies must be large—with at least 100,000 to 200,000 middle-age individuals—if they are to reliably measure end points in multiple population groups, within a 5- to 10-year period. These studies should focus on questionnaires and physical measurements. Biological sample collection may be included. Because prospective studies require rigorous follow-up over a number of years, they are best done when the required infrastructure and long-term research units are in place.

• **Systematic review of past epidemiologic studies** of CVD in developing countries may provide information useful for policy planning. Methodological advances in meta-analysis of observational studies may help develop useful data on the age-specific prevalence of CVD deaths and risk factors and on their trends. Since most of the earlier studies are small and not often found in computerized databases such as Medline, efforts to collate previous studies would rely on a combination of journal searches and contact with researchers. These systematic reviews could be a useful way to organize networks of researchers. Such approaches could also be applied to evaluations of past randomized trials, although few of these have been done in developing countries. Experience with meta-analysis of randomized controlled trials suggests that international collaborative efforts using original patient data provide more valid results. Finally, judicious use of hospital admission and discharge data could provide limited, but useful, information on the age, sex, and other characteristics of CVD cases.

After evaluating the respective strengths and limitations of the different analytic studies described above, the committee recommends that immediate support be directed to determining the morbidity and mortality of conventional and new risk factors for CVD and assessing their interactions through the use of incident case-control studies.

Public Health Interventions

Public health interventions are directed at entire populations or subpopulations. Appropriate research for these may range from randomized trials of the efficacy of treatment in individuals to quasi-random or other systematic evaluations at the community level to assess the effectiveness of interventions in actual-use situations.

Randomized Trials

Randomized trials are the best method for establishing the efficacy and magnitude of the impact of intervention on CVD control. Evidence from such trials has led to dramatic changes in the use of medications and the practice of cardiology in developed countries.

Randomized trials studying salt reduction through dietary guidance or substitution of potassium may be useful in populations with a high mortality from stroke. The proportion of hemorrhagic stroke is higher in developing country populations (Reddy and Yusuf, 1998). Since these events are known to be sensitive to blood pressure, even moderately successful interventions to reduce blood pressure could have a significant impact on CVD incidence.

Alternative applications of randomized trials would be to randomly assign clinicians or clinical sites to a package of interventions or an algorithm for CVD care (see below) and compare these with usual practice. Such trials could yield results that are generalizable and would be made more acceptable by the fact that they derive from studies directly involving the clinical community. Another possibility is to increase participation from developing countries in international trials of low-cost treatments.

Clinical Interventions

Essential Vascular Package

A wealth of evidence from randomized trials indicates that several clinical treatments can provide cost-effective care for established vascular patients. Aspirin, beta-blockers, ACE (angiotensin-converting enzyme) inhibitors, and cholesterol-lowering statin drugs reduce the probability of death and subsequent nonfatal, major vascular events in patients with established ischemic heart disease. However, to have a sustained effect in developing countries, these drug packages must be low cost and widely accessible. Although cholesterol-lowering drugs such as statins are currently expensive compared to aspirin or beta-blockers, their costs may decrease in the next 5 years when their patents expire. These would then be key components of the essential vascular package, or EVP. The committee considers that such an EVP could benefit large numbers of people in developing countries. Because its delivery relies on self-presentation it has no screening costs and could be highly cost-effective. Packaging EVPs into single, daily formulations could substantially improve compliance, as it did for treatment of tuberculosis.

The goals of the EVP should be (1) to select low-cost, generic versions of these drugs; (2) to achieve near-universal access; and (3) to price these packages so they are affordable for developing world clinics and patients. The EVPs should first be assessed for acceptability, use, and outcome to ensure their successful adoption. Such testing could be in the form of randomized trials that assess the EVP versus standard clinical care. If acceptable, the EVP should be included in a publicly financed, universally available package of clinical services and on insurance treatment lists. Efforts to educate physicians and increase patient awareness about the value of such packages should also be supported. The second and third goals of the EVP can be addressed by pricing reimbursements of treatments to the lowest-cost basis of the EVP.

In summary, the committee recommends that research be directed to the following:

• evaluating the responses of different ethnic populations to cardiovascular drugs and interventions, and their implications for rational drug treatment.

• expanding the participation of developing country centers in multicenter collaborative clinical trials of EVPs and other potentially affordable, widely applicable interventions.

Algorithms for Effective Diagnosis and Clinical Management

Algorithms for the clinical care of CVD could improve the awareness and use of effective treatments. To be maximally effective, they should be adapted to different cultural needs and be widely applicable and usable by nonphysicians and physicians for various levels of care. Each algorithm should define clinical diagnostic or presumptive criteria, along with the steps for administering and evaluating simple medical treatments. The algorithms should, at a minimum, address the following clinical problems:

1. treatment of acute coronary ischemia, acute stroke, and transient ischemic attack, chronic coronary ischemia, chronic peripheral vascular disease, and congestive heart failure;
2. management of low-cost, home-based rehabilitation following a stroke or myocardial infarction; and
3. guidelines on the detection and treatment of elevated blood pressure and on the screening and treatment of elevated cholesterol.

For each algorithm, it will be important to measure its acceptability and use, to determine how to market it to the public and private sectors, and to cooperate with the pharmaceutical industry in this process. Algorithms should be developed and implemented according to the local characteristics of disease, cultural norms, and health service settings. Monitoring the effects of algorithms on disease outcome is essential.

In summary, the committee recommends that research be undertaken to evaluate algorithms for the clinical diagnosis and affordable management of the following: (1) hypertension, (2) dyslipidemia, (3) diabetes, (4) acute myocardial infarction, (5) angina, (6) stroke, (7) transient ischemic attacks, (8) congestive heart failure, (9) peripheral vascular disease, (10) post-myocardial infarction rehabilitation and risk management, and (11) poststroke rehabilitation and risk management.

Randomized Trials of Other Low-Cost Treatments

There is growing evidence that homocysteine is a risk factor for coronary heart disease and that low-cost folate supplementation may reduce homocysteine levels and thus the risk of heart disease. Randomized trials assessing the cardiovascular benefit of folate supplementation are needed, and several trials are being planned or are under way in developed country populations. Since folate intake and blood levels among adults in developing countries are believed to be lower than those in industrial countries, randomized trials of this intervention should also be considered for developing country populations.

Inclusion of Developing Countries in International Collaborative Clinical Trials

The evaluation of lifesaving technologies through randomized clinical trials often involves collaboration among investigators in several countries with diverse populations. To date, however, these trials have been conducted primarily in developed countries. The inclusion of populations and scientists from developing countries in future trials will help to (1) extend the generalizability of trial results; (2) understand different ethnic responses to cardiovascular drugs and other interventions; (3) compare the cost-effectiveness of interventions in developing country populations; and (4) enhance research capacity.

Other Public Health Interventions

Many other issues of program effectiveness can be addressed through systematic demonstration studies designed to yield rigorous results through standardized evaluation and serial implementation in successive communities with comparable pre- and postevaluation strategies. Such approaches can address effects at the community (rather than the individual) level where random allocation of larger numbers of observational units may not be feasible, affordable, or acceptable.

RESEARCH TO CONTROL SPECIFIC RISK FACTORS

Research on CVD control should focus on the risk factors that contribute most to the current and projected burden of disease in developing countries. Such research has several goals:

• periodically estimate the rates or levels of exposure to a risk factor in the population;
• develop and validate cost-effective methods for identifying exposed individuals at high risk of CVD;
• assess the capacity of health care delivery systems to implement programs for the detection and control of these risk factors; and
• evaluate the cost-effectiveness of programs aimed at: reducing the population-wide risk, the risk to persons already at high risk, and the risk to persons who have clinically manifest CVD.

Attention should be given to selecting the risk factors for early intervention. These would include risk factors that contribute to more than one CVD or NCD. Knowledge of population-specific conditions can make such public health actions more effective.

The Global Burden of Disease Study identifies tobacco use and hypertension among the major risk factors contributing to the present and projected mortality and disability from NCDs (Murray and Lopez, 1997b). Interventions aimed at reducing the levels of tobacco use and hypertension in developing country populations deserve high priority.

Tobacco Use

Nearly three-quarters of the more than 1 billion people who regularly use tobacco live in developing countries (Jha, 1997). By the year 2030, tobacco is predicted to kill approximately 10 million people annually in developing countries, which is triple the current mortality caused by tobacco (Peto, 1997). In most developed countries, the epidemiologic transition described in Chapter 2 has been followed by a behavioral transition to unhealthy behaviors, including smoking. Because this transition has not occurred yet or has begun recently in some developing countries, it is still possible to stop the tobacco epidemic at an early stage.

As noted by the Institute of Medicine (IOM, 1998), "The success of tobacco control efforts in developed countries has largely been due to the cultivation of a receptive social and political climate through the availability of information about the real risks of tobacco use, supported by research on appropriate pricing and regulation." There is a similar need for developing countries to establish knowledge on the extent of tobacco-related CVD mortality; the determinants of tobacco use, including the impact of advertising, promotion, and price; the costs of tobacco use; and cost-effective strategies for reducing tobacco use. Local knowledge will allow for political, social, and cultural differences among developing country populations, while striving for comparability across studies.

Research on tobacco control can help reduce the substantial burden of disease projected for several tobacco-related diseases, including certain cancers and chronic obstructive pulmonary disease as well as CVD (see Chapters 1 and 2; CDC, 1990, 1994; WHO, 1997).

Thus, research on tobacco control in developing countries should be undertaken to (1) estimate the prevalence of regular tobacco use in population samples; (2) monitor tobacco consumption trends in especially vulnerable groups, such as children, adolescents, and women; (3) evaluate the cost-effectiveness of community-based intervention programs that promote abstinence from tobacco; (4) evaluate the cost-effectiveness of tobacco cessation programs aimed

at changing the behavior of current smokers; and (5) evaluate the economic impact of tobacco control on developing countries that grow, manufacture, or export tobacco products in order to encourage alternative crops.

Hypertension

High blood pressure is widely prevalent in developing countries and a major contributor to coronary heart disease and to hemorrhagic and thrombotic stroke. More than twice as many deaths from stroke occur in the developing countries as in the developed countries (see Chapters 1 and 2).

Even small changes in the population distribution of blood pressure can have a profound impact on CVD rates. In high-risk persons who have developed clinical hypertension, the benefits of blood pressure reduction through drug therapy are substantial. Evidence from clinical trials demonstrates that a 5–6 mm Hg reduction in diastolic blood pressure will reduce stroke death by 35–40 percent and coronary deaths by 15–20 percent (WHO, 1996a).

Hypertension control programs are an effective starting point for CVD prevention and control for the following reasons:

- hypertension is a risk factor for both coronary heart disease and stroke;
- such programs have a "clinical" appeal to both the care providers and the community;
- the goals are easily measurable;
- the impact on hypertension awareness, treatment status, and level of control can be measured in a relatively short time (five years);
- the programs provide a natural coalition of various categories of health care providers, each with an important role in the detection or management of hypertension and its sequelae; and
- the concept of "comprehensive cardiovascular reduction" as a part of hypertension management makes it possible to incorporate strategies aimed at modifying other CVD risk factors such as tobacco use, high blood lipids, diabetes, and obesity.

Thus, the committee recommends that research on hypertension control in developing countries be undertaken to:

- **estimate the distribution of elevated blood pressure and prevalence of hypertension in population samples;**
- **evaluate the cost-effectiveness of community-based, life-style-linked interventions such as improved nutrition and exercise, and reduced smoking to decrease the incidence of high blood pressure;**

    • **assess the cost-effectiveness of programs to detect and treat hypertension by improving awareness, treatment initiation and adherence, and level of control; and**
    • **evaluate the effectiveness of low-cost combination drug therapies developed by countries such as China.**

Diet and Physical Activity

Profound demographic changes are increasing the proportion of populations in middle- and older-age groups where adult CVD becomes common. In addition, as cultures adapt to become more "Western," diet and physical activity are adversely affected. Global R&D is needed to identify successful ways to "delink" social and economic development from adverse changes in diet and physical activity. These changes will determine in large part the course of the CVD epidemic (Labarthe, 1998).

HEALTH SERVICES RESEARCH

Review of Patterns of Clinical Practice

A systematic review of medical practice patterns should identify effective ways of diagnosing CVD and of treating it effectively. These reviews could be conducted in hospital settings in several countries, with standardized diagnostic methods. The CVD-related conditions to be included are acute coronary ischemia, acute stroke and transient ischemia, chronic coronary ischemia, chronic peripheral vascular disease, and congestive heart failure.

Research on CVD control should include consideration of the influence of professional training, prescribing behavior, and payment systems, such as prepayment versus fee for service on the treatments recommended. This would also review the influences on government decisions to fund hospital-based curative services versus population-based CVD prevention.

The Economic Burden and Cost-Effectiveness of Interventions

There are few data on the economic costs of CVD in developing countries. However, the rapid escalation in costs can be anticipated from the emerging epidemic of CVD (see Chapter 2). This could be a powerful motivation for policymakers to implement preventive CVD strategies. Studies addressing the economic burden caused by CVD in developing countries should focus on the effect of CVD on production, earnings, and household health. These studies will have to standardize definitions of cost across populations and among different health care systems. These studies could identify the costs borne by income group, sex, and rural or urban status.

There are limited data from developing countries on the effectiveness of CVD expenditures. Preliminary estimates from India suggest that population-based risk factor reduction and low-cost secondary treatments are as cost-effective as other interventions included in minimal essential packages of care (Jha et al., forthcoming). These studies should be incorporated into broader studies of the cost-effectiveness of medical care.

GOVERNMENT'S POLICY ROLE

There is a strong need for governments to review the policies guiding specific health interventions and to encourage evaluation of products and tools for their effectiveness. The role of government is to regulate, legislate, and provide information.

Tobacco Control Policy

The key elements of effective tobacco control are (1) setting high prices; (2) displaying serious and prominent health warnings on all tobacco products; (3) banning advertising and promotion of all tobacco-associated products or trademarks; (4) using cost-effective mass media to counter product advertising; (5) supporting research on the causes, consequences, and costs of smoking; (6) controlling smuggling; and (7) developing the capacity to monitor the burden of disease caused by tobacco and to lobby for tobacco control (IOM, 1998; Jha et al., forthcoming).

These policies were effective in reducing tobacco consumption by more than 40 percent in developed countries from 1960 to 1990 (Peto et al., 1994; World Bank, 1997b). Developing countries have not instituted effective tobacco controls and are projected to have a rapid increase in smoking. The problem is likely to be greatest in China, East Asia, South Africa, and the former Soviet states (Peto et al., 1994). National programs are needed to reduce current and future tobacco use.

Food and Nutrition Policy

The establishment of food and agriculture policies and nutrition goals has helped control consumption in developed countries of diets high in fat, sugar, and salt (Carleton et al., 1991; Grundy et al., 1997). These approaches can be effective in developing countries as well. The production, processing, packaging, labeling, and marketing of food items, as well as subsidies for their production, have to be assessed for their influence on dietary intakes. These goals should be coordinated with broad public health goals so that, for example, reducing salt consumption does not undermine programs for iodine supplementation through the use of iodized salt.

Pharmaceutical Policy

Provision by the health care system of low-cost pharmaceuticals for CVD treatment and the promotion of their rational use by health care providers require coordination of policies and practices in the manufacture, regulation, and pricing of pharmaceuticals, essential drug lists, and the influence of the pharmaceutical industry on prescribing practices.

Private-Sector Participation

The private sector can participate in population-based prevention programs, as well as in cost-effective case management programs. Partnerships with the private sector may also attract research funding to evaluate population-based interventions for risk factor modification and those testing clinical care algorithms.

BUILDING CAPACITY FOR RESEARCH AND DEVELOPMENT

To undertake research for the control of CVD in developing countries requires a strengthening of existing capacities for conducting research. This will require training investigators in (1) population-based epidemiologic research, (2) clinical research, (3) health policy research, and (4) economic evaluation of health care interventions. It will also require strengthening linkages among basic, epidemiologic, clinical, and policy research areas so that CVD can be targeted with a problem-solving, multidisciplinary approach.

There are programs that provide such training. The Scientific Council on Epidemiology and Prevention of the International Society and Federation of Cardiology (ISFC) conducts an annual seminar on CVD epidemiology and prevention for 30–35 international fellows drawn from diverse health disciplines. About one-third to one-half of these fellows are from developing countries. The International Clinical Epidemiology Network (INCLEN) has a training program for clinical researchers, social scientists, statisticians, and health economists from selected academic institutions in developing countries. Although it is not specifically directed to CVD-related research, this program has augmented the capacity for health research in developing countries through multidisciplinary and international collaboration. There are also formal training programs for epidemiologists and clinicians in various academic institutions are accessible through fellowship programs sponsored by governments, the World Health Organization (WHO), and international aid agencies.

More trained investigators are needed for CVD-relevant research. The unfinished health agenda of the developing world and the emergence of the HIV–AIDS epidemic have restricted the number of epidemiologists available to investigate CVD epidemiology. Nutritional research on NCDs has not engaged attention due to continuing and justified concerns about deficiency disorders. Clinical investigators have been more preoccupied with applications of high-technology interventions than with testing widely needed, low-cost, clinical algorithms for diagnosis and management of CVD.

Hence, there is a growing need to train individuals and equip institutions to undertake research relevant to CVD control. Regional training programs, modeled after the ISFC seminars and the INCLEN program, could be established in developing countries to focus on the control of CVD and other NCDs. Institutional capacity for conducting integrated, problem-oriented research could be strengthened with training and equipment for institutions that have the potential to undertake epidemiologic, clinical, and policy research.

Much of the research methodology already developed, tested, and applied can be transferred to developing countries. Agencies such as WHO can facilitate this process, both as a central repository of information and by providing subsidized pharmaceuticals. There are mutual benefits to be derived from twin-center programs between developed and developing countries. Regional research networks can effectively link institutions within and among developing countries to leverage scientific expertise and financial resources.

In summary, the committee recommends establishing or expanding the following capacity-strengthening capabilities in developing countries: (1) training programs in cardiovascular epidemiology, clinical research methodology, health policy research, and health economics; (2) the institutional capacity for undertaking integrated research relevant to CVD control; and (3) channels of collaboration through twin-center programs and regional research networks.

6

◆ ◆ ◆ ◆ ◆

Institutional Arrangements for
Research and Development

International research on cardiovascular disease (CVD) has a history of four decades or more and includes the CVD Unit of the World Health Organization (WHO), the International Society and Federation of Cardiology (ISFC) with its scientific councils and Section on Epidemiology and Prevention, and specific efforts initiated in several developed countries over the same period. International collaboration has been encouraged by the ISFC's sponsorship of the International Conferences on Preventive Cardiology (ICPC) every four years. These were held in Moscow in 1985; Washington, D.C., in 1989; Oslo in 1993; and most recently, Montreal in 1997. The growing participation of developing country scientists—reaching more than 400 of the nearly 3,000 registrants in 1997—demonstrates a widening recognition of the global dimensions of CVD. This recognition has led to a growing number of collaborations between institutions in developed countries and developing countries.

In addition to WHO and ISFC, national and international organizations engaged in CVD prevention and control include the International Clinical Epidemiology Network (INCLEN); United Nations Scientific, Educational and Cultural Organization (UNESCO); national and regional foundations; national academies of science and medicine in developed and in developing countries; medical schools and other academic centers of excellence; the World Bank; and donor agencies such as the Canadian International Development Centre and Swedish International Development Agency. Also, several networks have been established for the conduct of multinational randomized clinical trials in CVD, such as the International Studies of Infarct Survival (ISIS), Long Term Intervention with Pravastatin in Ischemic Disease (LIPID), and Global Utilization of

Streptokinase and t-PA (tissue plasminogen activator) for Occluded Coronary Arteries (GUSTO), among others.

Research on CVD has gradually expanded through the International Ten-Day Seminars on the Epidemiology and Prevention of CVD, sponsored by the ISFC with participation from WHO; U.S. and other national programs; and other short courses. The submission of nearly 1,500 scientific abstracts for the fourth ICPC in Montreal demonstrates the growth in CVD research. Several developing countries now have a critical mass of qualified health professionals to meet the challenges of the global CVD epidemic. In many others, however, the trained scientists and infrastructure are too few to address already urgent tasks.

It has become increasingly important to consider the organizational arrangements under which CVD prevention and control around the world can best be facilitated. This chapter outlines the need for appropriate institutional arrangements and identifies the functional requirements for achieving global CVD prevention and control. Based on these considerations and examples of successful models, the chapter concludes by proposing an immediate and long-term answer to the question, *How can global R&D for cardiovascular health best be institutionalized?*

Formal institutional arrangements for R&D in cardiovascular health are important for three reasons:

1. Many organizations and programs are engaged in activities relevant to CVD prevention and control. The impact of their work can be enhanced, and duplication avoided by effective exchange of information on CVD activities.

2. Activities in new and existing programs can be strengthened through a central agency that provides communication, coordination, and technical and material support.

3. A widely recognized central agency is needed to advocate for CVD prevention, to set R&D priorities, and to acquire and allocate resources to meet R&D priorities.

EFFECTIVE RESEARCH AND DEVELOPMENT AT LOCAL OR NATIONAL, REGIONAL, AND GLOBAL LEVELS

The immediate goal for cardiovascular R&D is to enhance local capacity through education and training; development of networks where appropriate; and conduct of local research that is comparable with other centers and applicable internationally. For activities in CVD prevention and control to be successful, it is essential that nonhealth sectors—for example, education, agriculture, industry, and environment—are also included in development of the program. Potential partnerships should be identified and integrated into the action plan.

The major functions to be undertaken at different levels are as follows:

1. **Local or National:** Develop and maintain the capacity and resources to plan, implement, and evaluate research and demonstration projects for CVD prevention. These should include:

- community-based assessment of the CVD burden;
- monitoring of and intervention in risk factors and their determinants;
- testing clinical interventions (e.g., EVP and algorithms for low-cost clinical care); and where feasible,
- investigating the local determinants of CVD risk.

2. **Regional:** Support local or national centers as they undertake their activities providing:

- technical support;
- communication and exchange of information;
- funding support from regional and international donors; and
- evaluation of the status of CVD prevention activities in the region.

3. **Global:** Support regional centers in the conduct of their activities:

- maintenance of global data on CVD prevention and control programs;
- dissemination of current data, protocols, guidelines, and literature on CVD prevention and control; and
- convening of advisory groups to assess global needs, evaluate current activities, and recommend additional activities if they are needed.

MODELS OF INTERNATIONAL COLLABORATION

International collaborations can be highly effective. Two of the most effective models are described here.

The Special Programme for Research and Training in Tropical Diseases

In 1975 the United Nation Development Programme (UNDP)–World Bank–WHO established a Special Programme for Research and Training in Tropical Diseases (TDR) to relieve the burden of tropical diseases around the world. In the 20 years since its establishment, TDR has been dramatically successful in its international partnerships, among the three cosponsoring agencies, with other organizations working in similar areas, and among the more than 5,000 scientists in 160 countries who collaborate in its activities. This model has several key characteristics:

- strong leadership;
- support of program staff;
- generous donations from cosponsors, bilateral development agencies, private foundations, and governments of some developing countries;
- emphasis on periodic performance evaluation; and
- management that emphasizes scientific priorities.

The MONICA Project

MONICA is the WHO Multinational *Moni*toring of Trends and Determinants in *Ca*rdiovascular Disease. This project complements the older cross-sectional studies of incidence of disease with additional longitudinal investigation of CVD determinants and outcomes. The MONICA project initiated the simultaneous monitoring of cardiovascular mortality, morbidity, case fatality, risk factor levels, and social and behavioral trends in defined communities. Over time these trends were used to identify causal relationships and interactions among variables. Because MONICA replicates the same core of observations in many different communities, the project is beyond the scope of any single research unit or national action. The model has accomplished the following favorable outcomes:

- a 10-year study in 60 countries in North America, Europe, and the former Soviet Union, along with Australia, New Zealand, China, Japan, and Malta;
- a common study protocol and centralized laboratory–electrocardiogram evaluation centers;
- a defined population for study within each center;
- census data defining each population by sex and age;
- population surveys at the beginning and end of the 10-year study period, which included at least 200 individuals in each 10-year age and sex group between ages 35 and 64; and
- collection of annual data on the use of health services by each population.

Additional examples illustrating successful national and international collaborations are cited in the supplement of the Catalonia Declaration (CDC, 1997). Collectively these examples illustrate strong potential for CVD prevention and control if well organized.

DEVELOPMENT OF AN INSTITUTIONAL MECHANISM FOR CARDIOVASCULAR RESEARCH AND DEVELOPMENT

An institutional mechanism is required for a sustained, global R&D that supports efforts for CVD prevention and control. To ensure prompt attention to the urgent needs in this area, the committee recommends that a Steering Committee for Cardiovascular R&D be established immediately under the aegis of the Global Forum for Health Research. The functions of this committee would include, but not be limited to, the following: (1) establishment of a program for competitive grants and setting of priority areas modeled after the UNDP–World Bank–WHO Special Programme for Research and Training in Tropical Diseases; (2) establishment of a global network on CVD health policy; and (3) promotion of financial and technical exchange among researchers and agencies or ministries of science and technology in industrialized countries, industries, and others.

The committee recommends that the activities of the steering committee be modeled after the TDR program with its broad range of participants that include scientists and donor agencies such as foundations, bilateral development agencies, and governments. Although the MONICA project is a strong model it was smaller, limited mainly to Europe and North America, lacked stable funding, and operated for a shorter term.

For the longer term, the committee recommends that WHO assume the lead in promoting global CVD control, adopting a TDR-like mechanism for this purpose. This recommendation is consistent with the view of international experts who attended the Fourth International Conference on Preventive Cardiology at Montreal in June 1997. Participants noted that for more than 30 years, WHO, through its Cardiovascular Disease Unit, has played a critical role in addressing major issues of global prevention and treatment. Although this role has been seriously curtailed in the recent past, the committee has concluded that a renewed commitment to CVD control by WHO offers the best prospect for establishing the necessary infrastructure to ensure sustained R&D in support of CVD prevention and treatment worldwide.

The two models proposed by the committee should seek to involve the professional component of cardiovascular medicine, which is currently organized globally into three intercontinental societies—European, InterAmerican, and Asian Pacific—under the umbrella of the International Society and Federation of Cardiology. This existing network of national professional societies and foundations is composed essentially of volunteers. As such, it currently lacks the funding, substantive infrastructure, and managerial capacity to be a realistic alternative to the models proposed here. However, this network could assist in providing appropriate scientific consultation, project review, and even project oversight for the primary body chosen.

Finally, it is worth noting that the Institute of Medicine in its recent publication *America's Vital Interest in Global Health* (IOM, 1997) defined "global health" as health problems, issues, and concerns that transcend national boundaries and that may best be addressed by cooperative action. Thus, the United States and other developed countries—in partnership with developing countries and with international organizations, industry, academia, foundations, and other nongovernment entities—must lead from their strengths in medical science and technology to play a central role in global health (see Appendix A for further rationale). Partnerships among countries and agencies are a key element for the cost-effective and sustained R&D that is needed to support global CVD control.

◆ ◆ ◆ ◆ ◆

Epilogue

This report addresses the question recently raised by the Institute of Medicine in *America's Vital Interest in Global Health* (IOM, 1997) and "The Pursuit of Global Health: Relevance of Engagement for Developing Countries" (Howson et al., 1998): *Why should countries in the developed world care about the emerging epidemic of cardiovascular disease (CVD) in developing countries?* The benefits of engagement have to be recognized if there is to be sustained international attention to the CVD epidemic.

ECONOMIC IMPACT

As the CVD epidemic emerges in developing countries, it has an increasingly severe impact on men and women in their productive middle years, as well as on those who are older. The growing middle class of many developing countries is experiencing the first phase of the CVD epidemic, which for many is disrupting family stability and family income. This has consequences for society as a whole. The cost of treatment can also have a serious impact on a country's health care expenditures and its economic development. For these reasons, development of effective approaches for CVD prevention and cost-effective management are urgent. Without effective prevention, the epidemic is predicted to expand, causing a profound impact on individuals and the country.

ETHICAL CONCERN: THE CONCEPT OF HEALTH FOR ALL

Developed countries were able to decrease mortality and morbidity from infectious diseases in the first half of the twentieth century because of the development of vaccines and other public health measures. They shared successful approaches and resources with developing countries through international assistance programs after World War II. There is a parallel opportunity for sharing knowledge on CVD prevention. Developed countries experienced an epidemic of CVD in the middle of this century and have since achieved a remarkable decline in cardiovascular mortality. Accomplishing this required major conceptual shifts in epidemiologic research (both observational and interventional), creation of a strong scientific database to guide policy and practice, and development of public information to discourage behaviors that predispose to CVD. As a similar epidemic of chronic diseases, especially CVD, emerges in developing countries, health professionals from developed countries are motivated to again share their experience of policies and approaches that have proven successful.

NATIONAL RELEVANCE

Worldwide immigration has created ethnic diversity in many countries such as the United States, Canada, Malaysia, and Singapore. Several studies from these countries indicate important differences in the incidence of CVD for recent immigrants now exposed to a new set of environmental risks. Some of these differences may be attributable to socioeconomic factors and culturally based patterns of diet, behavior, and activity, whereas others may be attributable to genetic factors. Studies of ethnically diverse groups in their original homeland and their newly adopted country continue to provide insights that improve understanding of the complexities and approaches for reducing the burden of CVD in the wider population.

SCIENTIFIC DISCOVERY

Studies addressing the development, prevention, and management of CVD in developing countries can contribute significantly to the overall knowledge base of CVD worldwide. The Framingham Heart Study and other developed country longitudinal studies identified key risk factors. However, considerable unexplained risk remains, and the relative importance of risk factors may differ among ethnic or socioeconomic groups and may change over time. The opportunity to study a new epidemic in different populations with different genetic characteristics, different exposures, and different cultural patterns can provide information that is broadly applicable.

Success in reducing CVD mortality in developed countries has been attributed to a wide range of strategies for prevention and treatment, including management of acute events. The relative contribution of preventive strategies remains unclear. With limited resources for management of acute events, developing country programs may provide a clearer picture of the contribution of prevention alone, or of prevention and low-cost treatment, in lowering the CVD burden. This knowledge would contribute significantly to policy and planning for all countries.

GLOBAL HEALTH ISSUES

Finally, the rapid spread of infectious diseases has emphasized the global nature of health risks. For CVD and other chronic diseases, policy changes in one country may have major effects on other countries. For example, tobacco regulations in the United States, Canada, and Australia have successfully decreased tobacco use in these countries. Tobacco manufacturing and promotion have intensified already in developing countries, While the burden of CVD is rapidly increasing, global surveillance and action are required to monitor changes in environmental and behavioral risks as CVD and other chronic diseases reach epidemic proportions. At the same time, health problems caused or exacerbated by tobacco use are likely to increase in developing countries as smoking becomes more prevalent there. As environmental and behavioral risks migrate internationally, they require global surveillance and action.

◆ ◆ ◆ ◆ ◆

References

Abraham, W.T., and Bristow, M.F. Specialized centers for heart failure management. *Circulation* 96:2755–2757, 1997.

Ad Hoc Committee on Health Research Relating to Future Intervention Options. *Investing in Health Research and Development.* Geneva: World Health Organization, 1996.

AHA (American Heart Association). *1993 Heart and Stroke Facts Statistics.* Dallas: American Heart Association, 1993.

AHA (American Heart Association). *Heart and Stroke Statistical Update, 1998.* Dallas: American Heart Association, 1998.

Azar, A.J., and Hofman, A. Costs and effects of long-term oral anticoagulant treatment after myocardial infarction. *Journal of the American Medical Association* 273:925–928, 1995.

Ballance, R., Pogany, J., and Gorstner, H. *The World's Pharmaceutical Industries. An International Perspective on Innovation, Competition and Policy.* Report prepared for the United Nations Industrial Development Organization (UNIDO). United Kingdom: Edward Elgar, 1992.

Barker, D.J.P., and Osmond, C. Infant mortality, childhood nutrition, and ischaemic heart disease in England and Wales. In Barker, D.J.P., ed., *Fetal and Infant Origins of Adult Disease.* London: British Medical Journal, 1992.

Barnum, H., and KutzIn J. *Public Health Hospitals in Developing Countries.* Published for the World Bank. Baltimore: The Johns Hopkins University Press, 1993.

Berrios, X., Koponen, T., Huiguang, T., Khaltaev, N., Puska, P., and Nissinen, A. *Distribution and Prevalence of Major Risk Factors of Noncommunicable Diseases in Selected Countries.* 75:99–108, 1997. Geneva: The World Health Organization Inter-Health Program.

Blackburn, H. The epidemiological basis of a community strategy for the prevention of cardiopulmonary diseases. *Annals of Epidemiology* S7:S8–S13, 1997.

Breslow, L. Social origins of cardiopulmonary disease: The need for population-focused prevention studies. *Annals of Epidemiology* S7:S4–S7, 1997.

Brownson, R.C., Koffman, D.M., Novotny, T.E., Hughes, R.G., and Eriksen, M.P. Environmental policy interventions to control tobacco use and prevent cardiovascular disease. *Health Education Quarterly* 22:478–498, 1995.

Bulatao, R., and Stephens, P. *Global Estimates and Projections of Mortality by Cause, 1970–2015.* Washington, D.C.: World Bank Population, Health, and Nutrition Department (PRE Working Paper 1007), 1992.

Carleton, R.A., Dwyer, J., Finberg, L., Flora, J., Goodman, D.S., Grundy, S.M., Havas, S., Hunter, G.T., Kritchevsky, D., Lauer, R.M., Luepker, R.V., Ramirez, A.G., Van Horn, L., Stason, W.B., and Stokes III, J.. Report of the expert panel on population strategies for blood cholesterol reduction. *Circulation* 83:2154–2232, 1991.

CDC (Centers for Disease Control and Prevention). *The Health Benefits of Smoking Cessation: A Report of the Surgeon General, 1990.* Washington, D.C.: U.S. Department of Health and Human Services, 1990.

CDC (Centers for Disease Control and Prevention). *Preventing Tobacco Use Among Young People.* Washington, D.C.: U.S. Department of Health and Human Services, 1994.

CDC (Centers for Disease Control and Prevention). *Worldwide Efforts to Improve Heart Health: A Follow-up to the Catalonia Declaration—Selected Program Descriptions.* Washington, D.C.: U.S. Department of Health and Human Services, 1997.

Cook, N.R., Cohen, J., Hebert, P.R., Taylor, J.O., and Hennekens, C.H. Implications of small reductions in diastolic blood pressure for primary prevention. *Archives of Internal Medicine* 155:701–709, 1995.

Cowie, M.R., Mosterd, A., Wood, D.A., Deckers, J.W., Poole-Wilson, P.A., Sutton, G.C., and Grobbee, D.E. The epidemiology of heart failure. *European Heart Journal* 18:208–225, 1997.

Cutler, J.A. Prevention of hypertension. Pp. 192–194 in *Hypertension Primer.* Dallas: American Heart Association, 1993.

Deubner, D.C., Tyroler, H.A., Cassell, J.C., Hames, C.G., and Becker, C. Attributable risk, population attributable risk, and population attributable risk fraction of death associated with hypertension in a biracial population. *Circulation* 52:901–908, 1975.

Dowse, G.K., Gareeboo, H., Alberti, K.G., Zimmet, P., Tuomilehto, J., Purran, A., Fareed, D., Chitson, P., and Collins, V.R. Changes in population cholesterol concentrations and other cardiovascular risk factor levels after five years of the noncommunicable disease intervention programme in Mauritius. Mauritius Non-Communicable Disease Study Group. *British Medical Journal* 311:1255–1259, 1995.

Enas, E.A., and Mehta, J.L. Malignant coronary artery disease in young Asian Indians: Thoughts on pathogenesis, prevention, and treatment. *Clinical Cardiology* 18:131–135, 1995.

Epsteln F.H. The relationship of lifestyle to international trends in C.H.D. *International Journal of Epidemiology* 18(3, Suppl. 1):S203–S209, 1989.

Forrester, J.S., Merz, C.N., Bush, T.L., Cohn, J.N., Hunninghake, D.B., Parthasarathy, S., and Superko, H.R. 27th Bethesda Conference: Matching the intensity of risk factor management with the hazard for coronary disease events. Task Force 4. Efficacy of risk factor management. *Journal of the American College of Cardiology* 27:991–1006, 1996.

Forsen, T., Eriksson, J.G., Tuomilehto, J., Teramo, K., Osmond, C., and Barker, D.J. Mother's weight in pregnancy and coronary heart disease in a cohort of Finnish men: Follow up study. *British Medical Journal* 315:837–840, 1997.

Fuster, V., Gotto, A.M., Libby, P., Loscalzo, J., and McGill, H.C. 27th Bethesda Conference: Matching the intensity of risk factor management with the hazard for coronary disease events. Task Force 1. Pathogenesis of coronary disease: The biologic role of risk factors. *Journal of the American College of Cardiology* 27:964–976, 1996.

Goldman, L., Benjamln S.T., Cook, E.F., Rutherford, J.D., and Weinsteln M.C. Costs and effectiveness of routine therapy with long-term beta-adrenergic antagonists after acute myocardial infarction. *New England Journal of Medicine* 319:152–157, 1988.

Goldman, L., Garber, A.M., Grover, S.A., and Hlatky, M.A. Cost effectiveness of assessment of and management of risk factors. *Journal of the American College of Cardiology* 27:1020–1030, 1996.

Gordis, L. *Epidemiology.* Philadelphia: W.B. Saunders Company, 1996.

Grabowsky, T.A., Farquhar, J.W., Sunnarborg, K.R., and Bales, V.S. *Worldwide Efforts to Improve Heart Health: A Follow-up to the Catalonia Declaration—Selected Program Descriptions.* Atlanta: Center for Disease Prevention and National Center for Chronic Disease Prevention and Health Promotion, 1997.

Grundy, S.M., Balady, G.J., Criqui, M.H., Fletcher, G., Greenland, P., Hiratzka, L.F., Houston-Miller, N., Kris-Etherton, P., Krumholz, H.M., LaRosa, J., Ockene, I.S., Pearson, T.A., Reed, J., Washington, R., and Smith, S.C., Jr. Guide to primary prevention of cardiovascular disease. A statement for healthcare professionals from the task force on risk reduction. *Circulation* 95:2329–2331, 1997.

Hanneman, R.L. INTERSALT: Hypertension rise with age revisited. *British Medical Journal* 312:1283–1284, 1996.

Howson, C.P., Bloom B.R., and Fineberg, H.V. The pursuit of global health: The relevance of engagement for developed countries. *Lancet* 351:586–590, 1998.

HSF (Heart and Stroke Foundation of Canada). *Cardiovascular Disease in Canada, 1993.* Ottawa: Heart and Stroke Foundation of Canada, 1994.

INTERSALT Cooperative Research Group. INTERSALT: An international study of electrolyte excretion and blood pressure: Results for 24-hour urinary sodium and potassium excretion. *British Medical Journal* 297:319–328, 1988.

IOM (Institute of Medicine), Board on International Health. *America's Vital Interest in Global Health.* Washington, D.C.: National Academy Press, 1997.

IOM (Institute of Medicine), National Cancer Policy Board. *Taking Action to Reduce Tobacco Use.* Washington, D.C.: National Academy Press, 1998.

Iso, H., Jacobs, D.R., Jr., Wentworth, D., Neaton, J.D., and Cohen, J.D. Serum cholesterol levels and six year mortality from stroke in 350,977 men screened for the multiple risk factor intervention trial. *New England Journal of Medicine* 320:904–910, 1989.

Jamison, D.T., Mosley, W.H., Measham, A.R., and Bobadilla, J.L., eds. *Disease Control Priorities in Developing Countries.* Oxford: Oxford Medical Publications, 1993.

Jha, P. International Implications of the Proposed U.S. Legal Settlement on Tobacco Manufacture, Production, and Marketing. Presentation at the National Cancer Policy Board Tobacco Control Workshop, Washington, D.C., July 15, 1997.

Jha, P., Jamison, D.T., and Habayeb, S. *Approaches to Control of Non-Communicable Disease in India, A World Bank Background Paper.* Washington, D.C.: World Bank, forthcoming.

Kannel, W.B., and Feinlieb, M. Natural history of angina pectoris in the Framingham study: Prognosis and survival. *American Journal of Cardiology* 29:154–163, 1972.

Kaplan, T., and Keil, J. Socioeconomic factors and cardiovascular disease: A review of the literature. *Circulation* 88:1973–1998, 1993.

Keil, U., and Kuulasmaa, K. WHO MONICA Project: Risk factors. *International Journal of Epidemiology* 18(3, Suppl. 1):S46–S55, 1989.

King, A.C., Jeffery, R.W., Fridinger, F., Dusenbury, L., Provence, S., Hedlund, S.A., and Spangler, K. Environmental and policy approaches to cardiovascular disease prevention through physical activity: Issues and opportunities. *Health Education Quarterly* 22:422–442, 1995.

King, H., Aubert, R.E., and Herman, W.H. Global burden of diabetes, 1995–2025: Prevalence, numerical estimates and projections. *Diabetes Care* (forthcoming).

KNA (Korean Neurological Association). Epidemiology of cerebrovascular disease in Korea. A collaborative study, 1989–1990. *Journal of Korean Medical Science* 8:281–289, 1993.

Krumholz, H.M., Cohen, B.J., Tsevat, J., Pasternak, R.C., and Weinstein M.C. Cost-effectiveness of a smoking cessation program after myocardial infarction. *Journal of the American College of Cardiology* 22:1697–1702, 1993.

Labarthe, D.R. *Epidemiology and Prevention of Cardiovascular Diseases: A Global Challenge.* Gaithersburg, MD: Aspen Publishers, Inc., 1998.

Law, M.R., Frost, C.D., and Wald, N.J. By how much does dietary salt reduction lower blood pressure? I. Analysis of observational data among populations. *British Medical Journal* 302:811, 1991.

Lowther, K.G., and Moonde, M.M. Planning, design and implementation of primary health care. *Experiences with Primary Health Care in Zambia.* Geneva: World Health Organization, pp. 15–26, 1994.

MacMahon, S., Peto, R., Cutler, J., Collins, R., Sorlie, P., Neaton, J., Abbott, R., Godwin J., Dyer, A., and Stamler, J. Blood pressure, stroke, and coronary heart disease. Part 1. Prolonged differences in blood pressure: Prospective observational studies corrected for the regression dilution bias. *Lancet* 335:765–774, 1990.

MacMahon, S., et al. Eastern stroke and coronary heart disease collaborative project, part 1: Methods and association of usual diastolic blood pressure with stroke and coronary heart disease in 124,774 individuals from 18 cohorts in Japan and the People's Republic of China, forthcoming.

Mahley, R.W., Palaoglu, K.E., Atak, Z., Dawson-Pepin J., Langlois, A.M., Cheung, V., Onat, H., Fulks, P., Mahley, L.L., Vakar, F., Ozbayrakci, S., Gokdemir, O., and Winkler, W. Turkish heart study: Lipids, lipoproteins, and apolipoproteins. *Journal of Lipid Research* 36:839–859, 1995.

Marmot, M.G., Smith, G.D., Stansfeld, S., Patel, C., North, F., Head, J., White, I., Brunner, E., and Feeney, A. Health inequalities among British social servants: The Whitehall II Study. *Lancet* 337:1387–1393, 1991.

Marques-Vidal, R., and Tuomilehto, J. Hypertension awareness, treatment and control in the community: Is the "rule of halves" still valid? *Journal of Human Hypertension* 11:213–220, 1997.

Martin J.D. Zambia—A country profile. see In *Experiences with Primary Health Care in Zambia.* Geneva: World Health Organization, pp. 1–6, 1994.

Mbanya, J.C., Ngogang, J., Salah, J., Minkoulou, E., and Balkau, A. Prevalence of NIDDM and impaired glucose tolerance in a rural and an urban population in Cameroon. *Diabetalogia* 40:824–829, 1997.

McGovern, P.G., Pankow, J.S., Shahar, E., Doliszny, K.M., Folsom, A.R., Blackburn, H., and Luepker, R.V. Recent trends in acute coronary heart disease—Mortality, morbidity, medical care, and risk factors. *New England Journal of Medicine* 334:884–890, 1996.

McKeige, P.M., Fenrie, J.E., Peirpont, T., and Marmot, M.G. Association of early-onset coronary heart disease in South Asian men with glucose intolerance and hyperinsulinemia. *Circulation* 88:152–161, 1993.

Michaud, C., Trejo-Gutierrez, J., Cruz, C., and Pearson, T.A. Rheumatic heart disease. In *Disease Control Priorities in Developing Countries*. New York: Oxford University Press, 221-223,1993.

Murray, C.J.L., and Lopez, A.D. *The Global Burden of Disease: A Comprehensive Assessment of Mortality and Disability from Diseases, Injuries, and Risk Factors in 1990 and Projected to 2020*. Boston: Harvard University Press, 1996.

Murray, C.J.L., and Lopez, A.D. Global mortality, disability, and the contribution of risk factors: Global burden of disease study. *Lancet* 349:1436–1442, 1997a.

Murray, C.J.L., and Lopez, A.D. Mortality by cause for eight regions of the world: Global burden of disease study. *Lancet* 349:1269–1276, 1997b.

Murray C.J.L., and Lopez A.D. Alternative projections of mortality and disability by cause, 1990–2020: Global burden of disease study. *Lancet* 349:1498–1504, 1997c.

Naylor, C.D., and Chen, E. Population-wide mortality trends among patients hospitalized for acute myocardial infarction: The Ontario experience, 1981 to 1991. *Journal of the American College of Cardiology* 24:1431–1438, 1994.

Neel, J.V. Diabetes mellitus: A thrifty genotype rendered detrimental by "progress"? *American Journal of Human Genetics* 14:353–362, 1962.

NHLBI (National Heart, Lung, and Blood Institute). Morbidity and mortality. *1996 Chart Book on Cardiovascular, Lung and Blood Diseases*. Washington, D.C.: National Institutes of Health, 1996.

Nissinen, A., Bothig, S., Granroth, H., and Lopez, A.D. Hypertension in developing countries. *World Health Statistics Quarterly* 41:141–154, 1988.

Olshansky, S.J., and Ault, A.B. The fourth stage of the epidemiologic transition: The age of delayed degenerative diseases. *Milbank Memorial Fund Quarterly* 64:355–391, 1986.

Omram, A.R. The epidemiological transition: A theory of the epidemiology of population change. *Milbank Memorial Fund Quarterly* 49:509–538, 1971.

Over, M., Ellis, R.P., Huber, J.H., and Solon, O. The consequences of adult ill-health. In *The Health of Adults in the Developing World*. New York: Oxford University Press, pp. 161–199, 1994.

Pasternak, R.C., Grundy, S.M., Levy, D., and Thompson, P.D. Spectrum of risk factors for coronary heart disease. *Journal of the American College of Cardiology* 27:978–990, 1996.

Pearson, T.A., and Fuster, V. Executive summary of the 27th Bethesda Conference. *Journal of the American College of Cardiology* 27:961–963, 1996.

Pearson, T.A., and Stone, E.J. Community trials for cardiopulmonary health: Directions for public health practice, policy, and research. *Annals of Epidemiology* S7:S1–3, 1997.

Pearson, T.A., Jamison, D.T., and Trejo-Gutierrez, J. Cardiovascular disease. In *Disease Control Priorities in Developing Countries*. New York: Oxford University Press, pp. 577–594, 1993.

Peto, R. Global Tobacco Mortality: Monitoring the Growing Epidemic. Presentation at the Tenth World Conference on Tobacco or Health, Beijing, China, August 24, 1997.

Peto, R., Lopez, A.D., Boreham, J., Thun, M., and Heath, C., Jr. *Mortality from Smoking in Developed Countries 1950–2000.* New York: Oxford University Press, 1994.

Pooling Project Research Group. Relationship of blood pressure, serum cholesterol, smoking habit, relative weight and ECG abnormalities to incidence of major coronary events: Final report of the Pooling Project. *Journal of Chronic Diseases* 31:201–306, 1978.

Reddy, K.S., and Yusuf, S. The emerging epidemic of cardiovascular disease in developing countries. *Circulation* 97:596–601, 1998.

Reed, D., and MacLean, C. The nineteen-year trends in C.H.D. in the Honolulu heart study. *International Journal of Epidemiology* 18(3, Suppl. 1):S82–S87, 1989.

Reed, D.M. The paradox of high risk of stroke in populations with low risk of coronary heart disease. *American Journal of Epidemiology* 131:579–588, 1990.

Republic of Korea Ministry of Health and Welfare. *Budget of Ministry of Health and Welfare, Fiscal Year 1996.* Seoul: Republic of Korea Ministry of Health and Welfare, 1996.

Republic of Korea Ministry of Health and Welfare. *White Paper 1997.* Seoul: Republic of Korea Ministry of Health and Welfare, 1997.

Rich-Edwards, J.W., Stampfer, M.J., Manson, J.E., Rosner, B., Hankinson, S.E., Colditz, G.A., Willett, W.C., and Hennekens, C.H. Birth weight and risk of cardiovascular disease in a cohort of women followed up since 1976. *British Medical Journal* 315:396–400, 1997.

Rose, G. Causes of the trends and variations in C.H.D. mortality in different countries. *International Journal of Epidemiology* 18(3, Suppl. 1):S174–S179, 1989.

Ross, R. The pathogenesis of atherosclerosis: A perspective for the 1990s. *Nature* 362:801–809, 1993.

Ryan, T.J., Anderson, J.L., Antman, E.M., Braniff, B.A., Brooks, N.H., Califf, R.M., Hillis, L.D., Hiratzka, L.F., Rapaport, E., Riegel, B.J., Russell, R.O., Smith, E.E., Jr., and Weaver, W.D. A.C.C./A.H.A. guidelines for the management of patients with acute myocardial infarction. A report of the American College of Cardiology/American Heart Association Task Force on Practice Guidelines, Committee on Management of Acute Myocardial Infarction. *Journal of the American College of Cardiology* 28:1328–1428, 1996.

Second International Heart Health Conference. *The Catalonia Declaration: Investing in Heart Health.* Autonomous Government of Catalonia, Advisory Board of the Second International Heart Health Conference, 1995.

Smith, S.C. Jr., Blair, S.N., Criqui, M.H., Fletcher, G.F., Fuster, V., Gersh, B.J., Gotto, A.M., Gould, K.L., Greenland, P., Grundy, S.M., Hill, M.N., Hlatky, M.A., Houston-Miller, N., Krauss, R.M., LaRosa, J., Ockene, I.S., Oparil, S., Pearson, T.A., Rapaport, E., and Starke, R.D. Preventing heart attack and death in patients with coronary disease. *Circulation* 92:2–4, 1995.

SOLVD Investigators. Effect of enalapril on survival in patients with reduced left ventricular ejection fractions and congestive heart failure. *New England Journal of Medicine*, 325:293–302, 1991.

Stone, E.J., Pearson, T.A., Fortmann, S.J., and McKinley, J.B. Community-based prevention trials. Challenges and directions for public health practice, policy and research. *Annals of Epidemiology* S7:S113–S120, 1997.

Thelle, D.S. Coronary heart disease mortality trends and related factors in Norway. *Cardiology* 72(1–2):52–58, 1985.

Thom, T.J. International mortality from heart disease: Rates and trends. *International Journal of Epidemiology* 18(3, Suppl. 1):S20–S28, 1989.

UN (United Nations). *World Population Prospects: The 1994 Revision.* New York: United Nations, 1995.

United Republic of Tanzania. *Policy Implications of the Adult Morbidity and Mortality End of Phase 1 Report.* Dar es Salaam: Ministry of Public Health, 1997.

Vartiainen, E., Dianjun, D., Marks, J.S., Korhonen, H., Guanyi, G., Ze-Yu, G., Koplan, J.P., Pietinen, P., Guang-LIn W., Williamson, D., and Nissinen, A. Mortality, cardiovascular risk factors and diet in China, Finland, and the United States. *Public Health Reports* 106:41–46, 1991.

Whelton, P.K., Brancati, F.C., Appel, L.J., and Klag, M.J. The challenge of hypertension and atherosclerotic cardiovascular disease in economically developing countries. *High Blood Pressure* 4:36–45, 1995.

WHO (World Health Organization). *Diet, Nutrition, and the Prevention of Chronic Diseases: Report of a WHO Study Group.* Geneva: World Health Organization Technical Report Series, 1990.

WHO (World Health Organization). *Diet, Nutrition, and the Prevention of Chronic Diseases.* Geneva: World Health Organization Technical Report Series, 1992.

WHO (World Health Organization). *Hypertension Control.* Geneva: World Health Organization Technical Report No. 862, 1996a.

WHO (World Health Organization). *Tobacco or Health: First Global Status Report.* Geneva: World Health Organization, 1996b.

WHO (World Health Organization). *The World Health Report 1996: Fighting Disease Fostering Development.* Geneva: World Health Organization, 1996c.

WHO (World Health Organization). *The World Health Report 1997: Conquering Suffering Enriching Humanity.* Geneva: World Health Organization, 1997.

Wolf, P.A. Epidemiology of stroke. In *Primer in Preventive Cardiology.* Dallas: American Heart Association, pp. 67–81, 1994.

World Bank. *World Development Report 1993: Investing in Health.* New York: Oxford University Press, 1993.

World Bank. *Mauritius Health Sector Review.* Washington, D.C.: World Bank, 1997a.

World Bank. *Sector Strategy Paper. Health, Nutrition, and Population.* Washington, D.C.: World Bank, 1997b.

Zatonski, W. *Evolution of Health in Poland Since 1988.* Warsaw: Maria Sklodowska-Curie Cancer Center and Institute of Oncology, Department of Epidemiology and Cancer Prevention, 1996.

APPENDIX A

◆ ◆ ◆ ◆ ◆

Five Steps for Setting Research Priorities

STEP 1: DETERMINE THE SIZE OF THE CVD BURDEN

Although it is not surprising that cardiovascular disease (CVD) is the leading cause of death worldwide because of its predominance in developed countries, it is surprising that CVD ranked second as a cause of death in all developing countries in 1990, with its burden almost equal to that of the leading cause—lower respiratory infections (see Table A-1). In fact, given the falling rates of infectious and parasitic diseases and the increasing rates of CVD in developing countries, CVD was most likely the developing world's leading cause of death by the mid-1990s. If ignored, this epidemic will increase drastically in the coming years.

Not only is CVD the largest cause of mortality in older age groups and in men, it is also a very significant contributor to mortality in persons of economically productive ages (i.e., 30–69 years) and in women (see Table A-2). Evidence shows that in 1990, CVD contributed to three times as many deaths worldwide in 30- to 69-year-olds as did infectious and parasitic diseases. This is true for both men and women, and it is true for all regions of the world except Sub-Saharan Africa. In this region, the numbers of deaths from CVD and infectious or parasitic diseases were about equal in 1990, and it is possible that CVD will soon dominate mortality in this region as well. This burden of disease and death in the economically most productive age stratum has important consequences for health care resources and for the economy in general, as indicated in Chapter 2.

STEP 2: IDENTIFY THE REASONS FOR THE CVD BURDEN

Diseases affecting the circulatory system are present during all stages of a country's development. Whereas CVD has been the dominant cause of death in developed countries for more than half a century, it is also emerging as the

77

dominant disease in developing countries. Although evidence from developed countries demonstrates that the control of CVD can be approached with measurable benefit through interventions at the individual, community, and national levels, this knowledge and experience have yet to be systematically applied in developing country populations. Thus, one reason the CVD burden persists and will increase in developing countries is because the potential implementation of intervention programs is hampered by the lack of appropriate awareness of cost-effective CVD control options and by concerns that such investments may detract from investments in communicable disease control and childhood, maternal, and reproductive health.

TABLE A-1 Ten Leading Causes of Death for 1990

Rank	Developed Regions	Total Deaths (thousands)	Developing Regions	Total Deaths (thousands)
1	Ischemic heart disease	2,695	Lower respiratory infections	3,915
2	Cerebrovascular disease	1,427	Ischemic heart disease	3,565
3	Trachea, bronchus, and lung cancer	523	Cerebrovascular disease	2,954
4	Lower respiratory infections	385	Diarrheal diseases	2,940
5	Chronic obstructive pulmonary disease	324	Conditions arising during the perinatal period	2,361
6	Colon and rectum cancers	277	Tuberculosis	1,922
7	Stomach cancer	241	Chronic obstructive pulmonary disease	1,887
8	Road traffic accidents	222	Measles	1,058
9	Self-inflicted injuries	193	Malaria	856
10	Diabetes mellitus	176	Road traffic accidents	777
	Total deaths	10,912	Total deaths	39,554

SOURCE: Murray and Lopez, 1996.

Another reason for the persistence of the emerging epidemic of CVD in low- and middle-income populations in developing countries is their increasing adoption of behaviors and life-styles that are known to elevate CVD risk. As indicated in Chapter 2, evidence suggests that the prevalence of established CVD risk factors such as tobacco use, elevated blood pressure, high saturated fat intake, obesity, and diabetes is increasing in these populations. The increasing rates of cigarette smoking alone are expected to increase CVD deaths in developing countries more than 18-fold in the next 22 years. These data are projected in

Table A-3. By the year 2020, the number of CVD deaths attributable to tobacco use is expected to surpass 2.5 million annually.

A third reason for the emerging epidemic of CVD in developing countries is largely unavoidable: the aging of populations due to declining fertility and the reduction in infant and childhood mortality (see Chapters 1 and 2).

In summary, the emerging epidemic of CVD in low- and middle-income country populations can be attributed to demographic change, rapid adoption of life-styles and habits associated with elevated CVD risk, and lack of current investment in intervention programs directed to the reduction and prevention of CVD risk factors and to the treatment and control of existing cases.

STEP 3: EVALUATE THE ADEQUACY OF THE CURRENT KNOWLEDGE BASE

Although much is known in developed countries about the distribution and influence of major risk factors for CVD, and lessons in prevention and treatment continue to be learned, there is little experience in applying this rich base of knowledge to the populations of low- and middle-income countries. Data on the nature, extent, and trends in disease occurrence and prevalence of major CVD risk factors are lacking for most regions of the developing world.

TABLE A-2 Deaths (thousands) Due to CVD and to Infectious and Parasitic Disease (IPD) in 30- to 69-Year-Olds by Sex and Region—1990

Region	Men		Women	
	CVD	IPD	CVD	IPD
Established market economies	483	42	227	12
Formerly socialist economies	263	20	163	6
India	611	429	481	240
China	576	158	439	89
Other Asian and Pacific Island countries	289	147	226	140
Sub-Saharan Africa	183	215	211	228
Latin American and Caribbean countries	186	62	147	48
Middle Eastern Crescent	285	83	215	85
Worldwide	3,028	1,128	2,201	798

SOURCE: Murray and Lopez, 1996.

TABLE A-3 Estimated Number of CVD Deaths (thousands) Worldwide Attributable to Cigarette Smoking and Percentage of Total Estimated Global Deaths—1990, 2000, 2010, and 2020

	1990	2000	2010	2020
Deaths attributable to cigarette smoking	955	1,399	1,931	2,613
Percentage of total deaths	1.9	2.5	3.2	3.8

SOURCE: Ad Hoc Committee on Health Research Relating to Future Intervention Options, 1996.

As a result, little is known about differences in CVD risk factors, clinical presentation, and outcomes in most developing world populations. Such differences may reflect variations in the prevalence of major established risk factors such as cigarette smoking, high blood pressure, hypercholesterolemia, and obesity, and possibly in the genetic predisposition to these risk factors. They may also reflect variations in unidentified risk factors. If governments and health providers are to respond adequately to the challenge of the emerging epidemic of CVD in developing countries, the committee believes they will need reliable data on the current and projected burden of CVD in their regions, as well as information on what they can do to reduce it. Many of the recommendations in this report, therefore, focus on epidemiologic data needs and on assessing the applicability of established CVD interventions in developing country populations. Such knowledge can be of critical importance, either confirming that approaches used elsewhere can be applied effectively or demonstrating that adaptation will be required.

STEP 4: EVALUATE THE PROMISE OF R&D EFFORTS

As Chapters 1 and 2 demonstrate, epidemiologic studies in developed countries provide abundant evidence for the preventability of CVD. In general, two broad strategies have been employed for CVD prevention in developed countries, namely, the high-risk approach and the population (public health) approach. The high-risk approach seeks to identify those with high levels of CVD risk factors and to treat these high-risk individuals intensively to reduce their risk. Although this approach can be effective for the individuals identified, it has limited the opportunity to reduce the population-wide burden of disease, since the large number of cases is not found in the small proportion at highest risk, but rather in those nearer the center of the distribution. Therefore, the population approach proposes to shift the entire distribution of CVD risk factors toward lower risk, so that substantial reduction of the overall population risk can be realized. Depending on circumstance (see Chapter 2), both strategies can be effective and many developed country populations use a combination of high-risk and population strategies.

Prevention strategies can be further divided into three categories from the perspective of risk factors: (1) "primordial prevention" is directed toward prevention of the risk factors themselves; (2) "primary prevention" focuses on reducing the existing risk factors (e.g., lowering blood pressure or the prevalence of cigarette smoking); and (3) "secondary prevention" is directed toward early detection and management of existing clinical disease (e.g., guidelines for management of acute myocardial infarction or heart attack).

Although primordial prevention strategies directed toward modifiable risk factors such as cigarette smoking, hypertension, and obesity have been shown to be effective in developed country populations, they have yet to be systematically investigated in developing countries but offer promise as cost-effective approaches. For its part, primary prevention of CVD—which has been shown in developed countries to be effective in randomized trials for elevated low-density lipoprotein (LDL) cholesterol, high-fat or cholesterol diets, hypertension, and especially cessation of cigarette smoking—should be assessed in developing world populations, particularly when low-cost interventions are sought or high-risk subgroups are targeted. Secondary prevention or case management strategies have been investigated extensively in patients in developed countries during both acute events and later phases of coronary heart disease and cerebrovascular disease. Interventions range from relatively inexpensive steps, such as behavioral risk factor control strategies (e.g., smoking cessation, lipid-lowering diet, physical activity, and weight reduction), to more expensive forms of technology (e.g., lipid-lowering drugs, aspirin, beta-blockers, and estrogens), to much more expensive technologies (e.g., thrombolytic therapies, automated internal defibrillators, coronary angiography with or without angioplasty and/or stent placement, coronary bypass surgery, cardiac transplantation).

Experience in developed country settings shows that effective interventions need not be costly. For example, marked improvements in survival from acute myocardial infarction after 1980 were largely due to the increasing use of aspirin, low-cost beta-blockers, and to a lesser extent, newer and more expensive clot-dissolving drugs. As indicated in Chapter 2 (Table 2-3), the relatively low-cost combination of aspirin and beta-blockers alone could prevent more than 210,000 deaths annually due to ischemic heart disease (IHD) and stroke in developing countries by the year 2020.

In summary, although many interventions with behavioral and inexpensive technologies are highly cost-effective in case management in developed countries, there is a need to assess the feasibility and cost-effectiveness of these management strategies in developing country settings. This same need extends to proven primordial and primary prevention approaches.

STEP 5: ASSESS THE ADEQUACY OF THE
CURRENT LEVEL OF EFFORT

Chapters 3 and 4 of this report address current patterns of CVD prevention and care and current levels and types of supporting R&D in developing countries. The message of these chapters is clear and consistent: few international donors or developing country governments recognize the importance of the emerging CVD epidemic in the developing world. In addition, in the majority of countries that have taken initial steps to address the epidemic, the focus has been on technology development, including building and supporting urban care facilities for diagnosis and treatment of CVD. There is little to no emphasis on developing, assessing, or implementing interventions for primordial and primary prevention in developing world populations. In the very few instances where developing country governments have emphasized prevention—see, for example, the successful case study of Zambia cited in Chapter 3—the resulting health benefits have been profound.

The committee's recommendations represent a synthesis of the evidence presented in this report and a distillation of the more numerous recommendations detailed in Chapter 5. The committee hopes that these recommendations will result in prompt and effective action to control CVD in developing countries, and that this action will be assisted by the Forum on International Health R&D and by other international donors, national governments, and professional organizations. The potential health and economic benefits of effectively engaging in the global fight against CVD are many. To continue as is, with the current inadequate level of effort, invites significant peril. An alternative future is possible, in which developing countries invest early enough to prevent the enormous costs of a major epidemic of CVD such as that experienced by developed countries in the twentieth century.

♦ ♦ ♦ ♦ ♦

Glossary of Cardiologic and Epidemiologic Terms

CLINICAL MANIFESTATIONS OF ATHEROSCLEROTIC CARDIOVASCULAR DISEASE

Manifestations of atherosclerotic disease may vary due to differences in risk factors and possibly genetic disposition. Atherosclerotic disease in the coronary arteries manifests itself as angina pectoris (40 percent), myocardial infarction (40 percent), and sudden cardiac death (20 percent) (Kannel and Feinlieb, 1972).

Angina pectoris: Condition due to the narrowing of one or more coronary arteries by atherosclerotic plaques, so that physical exertion, emotion, et cetera, lead to increased cardiac demands for coronary blood flow, which cannot be met, producing symptoms of ischemia such as chest tightness.

Atherothrombotic stroke: Condition that results from the occlusion of one or more cerebral arteries leading to necrosis of the brain tissue dependent on the blood flow. This may lead to transient (reversible ischemic neurological deficit) or permanent loss of neurologic function. Most frequently, it is due to embolization of the atherosclerotic plaque or the thrombus forming on it (i.e., breaking off of material in the aorta, carotid, or vertebral arteries with material floating downstream until it lodges in one of the smaller cerebral arteries).

Myocardial infarction: Condition usually due to the total thrombotic occlusion of a coronary artery at the site of an ulcerated atherosclerotic plaque, leading to cessation of blood flow to a portion of the myocardium and subsequent necrosis of the ischemic myocardium. Case fatality rates for myocardial infarction vary but generally are about 30–35 percent in community-wide studies.

Peripheral arterial disease: The presence of atherosclerosis in the aorta and arteries of the lower extremities can cause inadequate blood flow during exercise, leading to a cramp-like pain called intermittent claudication. Weakening of the aortic wall by atherosclerosis can result in aortic aneurysm formation and rupture, which lead to cardiovascular collapse.

Sudden cardiac death: Death may be due to a massive myocardial infarction but may also be attributable to myocardial ischemic attack, which allows the establishment of arrhythmias characterized by rapid rates and a collapse of cardiac output.

Diseases That May Be Due to Effects of Hypertension on the Cardiovascular System

Hemorrhagic stroke: Neurologic deficit caused by the bursting of an intracerebral artery. The disruption of brain tissue and increase in cranial pressure are often fatal and almost always disabling.

Hypertensive heart disease: Condition in which the heart muscle initially increases in mass due to increase in work against elevated arterial pressure in the aorta. Eventually, the heart may become stiff and unable to fill with blood, or it may dilate with loss of myocardial cells, leading to congestive heart failure.

CARDIOVASCULAR RISK FACTORS

A variety of factors have been identified as possibly causative of atherosclerosis and its clinical sequelae. These risk factors can be classified as modifiable or not modifiable. Among modifiable risk factors, the evidence supporting their modification as a way to prevent cardiovascular disease (CVD) can be classified as established, likely, or unproven (Pasternak et al., 1996; Pearson and Fuster, 1996).

Risk factors for which modification has been shown in epidemiologic studies or clinical trials to reduce risk include *cigarette smoking,* increase in *low-density lipoprotein (LDL) cholesterol level* (the fraction that carries most of the cholesterol in the blood), *a high-fat and high-cholesterol diet, hypertension* (high blood pressure, usually defined as >140/90 mm Hg), *hypertrophy of the left ventricle* (thickening of the cardiac muscle, usually due to high blood pressure), and *thrombogenic factors* (as evidenced by reduced clinical cardiac events with treatment by aspirin or anticoagulants).

A number of other risk factors have good epidemiologic evidence for their association with CVD, but weaker evidence from clinical trials. These include *diabetes mellitus* (a metabolic syndrome that includes elevated blood sugar levels), *physical inactivity,* low levels of *high-density lipoprotein (HDL) cholesterol* (the lipoprotein fraction thought to be responsible for removing cholesterol from the arterial wall), *triglycerides* (another form of fat carried in the blood), obesity, and *postmenopausal status* in women. With the advent of additional clinical trial data, these risk factors are likely to join those that are considered established.

A number of other risk factors are being investigated for their association with CVD. These include *psychosocial factors* such as hostility and postinfarction depression; *lipoprotein(a)* (a lipid with both atherogenic and thrombogenic properties); *homocysteine* (a metabolite that may be elevated in blood); *oxidative stress* (an increase in free radicals [e.g., in cigarette smoke] or lack of an antioxidant such as vitamin E); and *lack of alcohol consumption* (research indicates that one to two drinks of alcoholic beverage per day reduce CVD risk over that of abstinence).

The final group of risk factors that appears to be nonmodifiable *includes age, male gender, low socioeconomic status* (heart disease in developed countries is associated with poverty), and *family history* of CVD at <55 years of age in male relatives and <65 years in female relatives.

EPIDEMIOLOGIC TERMS AND CONCEPTS[*]

Age adjustment: Process by which a standard age distribution is used to calculate rates so that observed differences cannot be due to age differences in the population.

Attributable risk: Amount or proportion of disease incidence that can be attributed to a specific exposure or risk factor.

Case fatality rates: Number of individuals dying during a specified time after the diagnosis of disease, divided by the number of individuals with the specific disease.

Disability-adjusted life years (DALY): Combination of life years lost due to premature mortality and years lived with disability adjusted for severity (Murray and Lopez, 1997b).

Incidence: Ratio of the number of new cases of the disease occurring in a population during a specified time to the number of persons at risk for developing the disease during that period.

Mortality rates: Total number of deaths in one year divided by the number of persons in the population at mid-year.

Population-attributable risk fraction: Proportion of disease incidence in the total population that can be attributed to a specific exposure or risk factor.

Prevalence: Ratio of the number of cases of disease present in a population at a specified time to the number of persons in the population at the time specified.

Primary prevention: Prevention of the development of disease in a person who does not have the disease.

---

[*]The following terms are based on Gordis (1996).

Primordial prevention: Prevention of the development of risk factors for a disease.

Proportionate mortality: Number of deaths from a single disease in a population at a specified time divided by total deaths in the population at that time.

Relative risk: Ratio of the risk in persons exposed to a risk factor divided by the risk in persons not exposed to the risk factor.

Secondary prevention: Prevention of recurrence of a disease in a person who has already been diagnosed with the disease.

Tertiary prevention: Prevention of disability, poor quality of life, and death in persons with advanced stages of a disease.

Years of life lost (YLL): Number of life years lost prior to a given age of expected survival, usually 65 years.